Touched

by

Breast Cancer

Stories of Courage and Hope

compiled by
Trish Springsteen

Touched by Breast Cancer

Compiled by Deborah Fay and Trish Springsteen
Edited by Snowflake Productions
Copyright © 2018 MJL Publications
First published 2018

Publisher: MJL Publications
              17 Spencer Avenue
              Deception Bay QLD 4508
              Australia
              www.mjlpublications.com.au

Each of the contributing authors in this book retain the rights to their individual contributions, all of which have been printed as a part of this compilation with their permission. Each author is responsible for any opinions expressed within their own stories.

ISBN# 978-0-6484221-0-5

Table of Contents

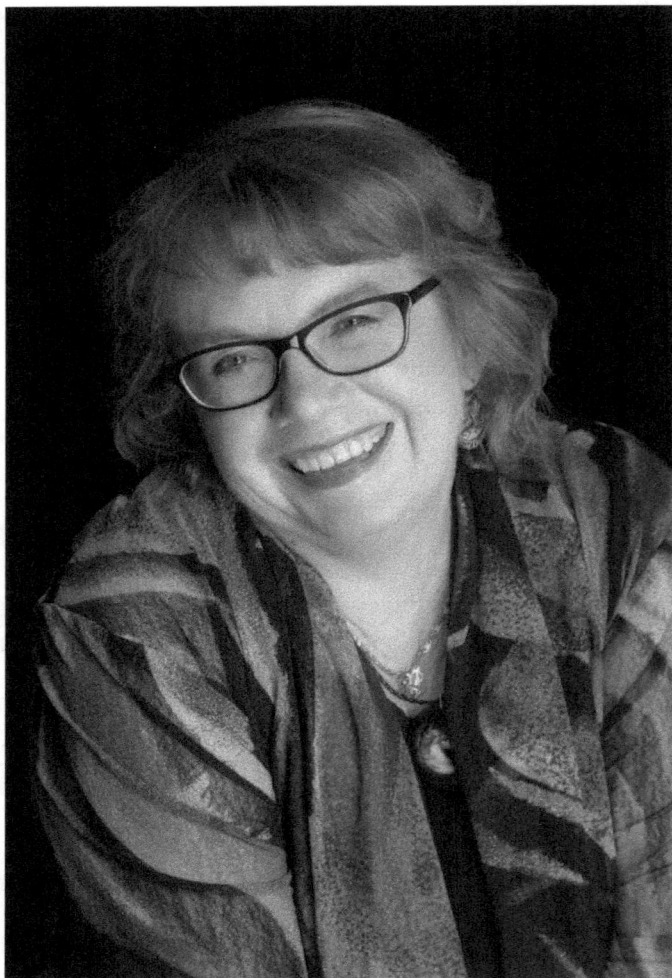

Introduction
By Trish Springsteen

February 2014 was the day I heard the words no-one wants to hear – "You have breast cancer!". I was alone, disbelieving and I remember my first reaction and words were, "I can't even win the Lotto and you are telling me I've got breast cancer?" Illogical response, I know, however when your whole life is about to be turned upside down your reactions can certainly come from left field.

So, what brought me to this day? Serendipity, actually, and one of the reasons I really, really like my General Practitioner. We had moved house a few months before and in the hassle I had not given my new address to the Breast Screening Clinic. It had been a couple of years since my last screening and it was not on my radar of people to notify with address change. Consequently, I never received my reminder for the screening. By pure luck that February I had a GP appointment for a minor issue, and while we were talking my doctor asked, "When did you have your last screening?" It was a throw-away question that was to have a tremendous impact on my life. I stopped and realised that I had not received my reminder – thanked him and immediately booked in for a regular screen check.

Off I went, had the screen, and was asked to come for a biopsy. I still wasn't worried. I'd had no symptoms, could feel no lump and I'd had a call back once before with no issues, just fatty tissue, so I hadn't asked anyone to come with me. So, there I was at Nambour Hospital having had the biopsy and was waiting for the results. I guess there may have been an inkling of worry when the doctor and the nurse walked in to the room. Then they dropped the bombshell. I really don't remember too much of that conversation – it was pretty much a blur. I do remember standing outside thinking, I have to hold this together, I've got to drive back home and it's a 40-minute drive on the highway. I'm supposed to stop in and see my mum on the way back, should I tell her? How could I do that, I need to speak to my husband first – do I ring him and tell him on the phone or just go straight home? You can see I really wasn't tracking too well. I went straight home and shared the news with my husband, rang my mum, contacted my daughter, let me sister and a couple of my long-time friends know and then just sat there trying to process all the emotions and feelings.

Thankfully, the Nambour people gave me written information and instructions – I contacted my GP, saw him straight away, he recommended a surgeon, and here serendipity strikes again – I was immediately able to get in to see her in 2 days as there had been a cancellation.

Now, I'm still not sure if what happened next was a good thing or not. It was a real whirlwind. After seeing the surgeon, I was booked in for surgery in 2 weeks. There wasn't any time for me to really stop and think and absorb everything. It just happened, one step after another. I had my own business, so was able to work things around that.

There I was in hospital having this weird procedure where they inserted wires so they could clearly identify lymph nodes and precise area – very futuristic look. Then it was up to the theatre for the surgery. Was I scared? What were my thoughts? To be honest, I believe I was still numb – it just all seemed to be happening in a blur.

Post-surgery and I am awake, waiting to hear the results. I'm lucky – picking up the cancer so early has given a good result – no spread – only a few lymph nodes out and partial breast. It could have been very much worse if I hadn't gone and had that screening test. Even better, the risk factors are good – no chemotherapy, just six weeks of radiation therapy. Every day for six weeks!

It was a long trek back and forth. The whole procedure was rather fascinating, a bit boring and rather cold laying there. At least now I can legitimately say I have three tattoos. Okay, they are three blue dots, however they are still tattoos. There is a silver lining in everything, you just have to look for it and decide how you are going to approach life.

I continued to run my business, do presentations and workshop whilst doing the radiation treatment. Was it tiring? Absolutely! Actually, you don't realise just how tired you are getting until you start to nod off at inconvenient times or find you can't get that usual enthusiasm to go to another network meeting or an event. I really didn't say too much about the whole diagnosis or the treatment at that time – I was just focusing on getting through this step, then the next, and the next.

I was often told, "You seem to be taking this all very well, with a good attitude." Well, you see, this actually wasn't the biggest life altering change that I had had in my life. In 2007, we lost our son Craig to suicide. So, my benchmark for acceptance, attitude and crisis was really high. Breast cancer for me was just something to get through, another curve life had thrown at me; however, compared to losing our son – well there was no comparison in terms of pain, confusion, life changing, grief, support and getting on with life. Was I upset, was I worried about the future, was I worried about the next five years and how I looked? Yes, yes and yes. It was just that there was no time to moan, to be down, to be negative. I got on with getting through this doing the best I could and was determined to have the best outcome I could.

Today, I am four and half years post – been taking tablets every day for the last four and half years, doctors' visits (three of them – a wonderful team, one of whom, Dr Rick Abraham, has been awesome to contribute to this book), bone density scans and blood tests. The side effects of the tablets have not been pleasant – menopause symptoms with hot flushes and sweating. That was really a pain as having had an endometrial ablation some years early I had thought I was going to avoid all those symptoms. My bone density started as being brilliant, as good as a 25-year-old athlete, which allowed me to start on the tablets that gave less side effects – except as the years have passed my bone density has reduced and reduced. So much so that in this last year I have had to change my tablets and these ones – well let's say I'm not too happy with some of the side effects. Only seven months to go – not that I am counting the days or anything. Seven months until I get the all clear and I can stop the tablets, the scans, the blood test and the doctor visits.

Am I still tired? Yes. Has it impacted my life? Yes. Has it impacted my business? Yes. Most importantly, has it impacted those around me? Yes.

Everyone handles crisis situations differently. Some hide, some deny, some are angry, some step up and others are inspirational. In all cases, we do not handle in isolation. What we have causes many ripples in our family, our friends and those around us.

For me, breast cancer has touched my sister, bringing the possibility to front of mind. She now has a family member with a history. It has touched my daughter – she too now has a family member with a history of breast cancer. It has touched my business. I found that the speaking skills that I have learnt in my business helped me to have the confidence to do a promotional interview on the breast screening site. Something I am passionate about because, for me, the early detection gave me a great result. It is something I share with clients, highlighting how speaking skills can help you in advocacy.

When I look back on the past four and a half years, I watch the ripples and the people that are touched by breast cancer. Those who get it, those who survive, those who don't, those who stand up and speak, those who quietly fundraise and support. The doctors faced every day by the reality of how much they can help, the nurses who work with those doctors.

The alternative healers who some people approach looking for another way to work through the situation. The not-for-profit organisations who support patients with breast cancer pillows and assistance in many ways. The tattooist who helps to reframe the outcome of mastectomies and the people who make the prosthesis and the bras.

So very many people touched in small and big ways! That is where the idea of this book came from. The concept was to invite people who have been touched by breast cancer to share their stories.

My hope is that you, the reader, will let these stories touch you, and through you, as you pass them on, touch others. There are messages of hope, information, and just people taking the opportunity to share their own story.

Please read, digest and allow yourself to be touched, changed and uplifted.

My thanks to Deborah Fay, MJL Publications, for supporting this book and assisting with sourcing the stories and keeping us on track.

As always, thanks to my husband, Peter, who has been there with me all through this journey, my rock, always supporting and always being the wind beneath my wings. He, too, has been touched and changed by this journey.

Thanks also to my wonderful family, my mother, my sisters, my brothers and my daughter, and to my long-time close friends, who have all supported and been there for me. This journey has touched you and your families as well.

Thanks to my four doctors, General Practitioner Dr Mark Zischke, Surgeon Dr Melinda Cook, Radiation Oncologist Dr Liz Kenny and Medical Oncologist Dr Rick Abraham. You have been a wonderful team who have never been too busy to answer questions. Each and every day you are touched by breast cancer.

Enjoy the book, take time to reflect and share. Live each day to the fullest as you never, never know what the new day will bring. However, live in light and happiness, not fear and doubt. Don't let the unknown pull you down – life is an adventure.

Be prepared – listen to your body, don't hide behind "it will never happen to me", because one day it just might.

Trish Springsteen is Australia's leading expert in empowering introverts, a multi international award-winning speaker mentor, international bestselling author and radio host. Clients work with Trish because they know she can help them have the confidence and self-belief to make speaking easy. Typically, Trish mentors introverts, authors and advocates helping them to share their message with those who need to hear it.

Trish Believes in You until You Believe in Yourself.

Trish has brought improved speaking and communication skills to published authors, advocates, bloggers and introverts. As well as communication, speaking and presentation skills to accountants from Crosbie Warren Sinclair; executives from The IQ Business Group and Aurecon; scientists from Rio Tinto Alcon; engineers from James Hardy and property retail experts from Jones Lang LaSalle.

Trish is the author, co-author and/or contributing author of 12 books and is featured in Motivational Speakers Australia.

www.trishspringsteen.com

info@trischel.com.au

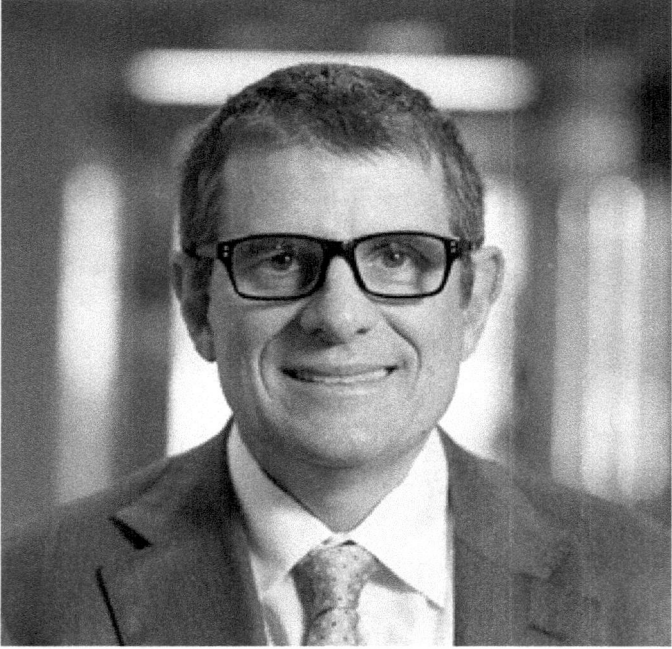

First Story

By Dr. Rick Abraham

I am a medical oncologist, or chemotherapy specialist, having initially worked as a fulltime "academic" oncologist at a large teaching hospital before embarking upon a pure private oncology practice more than a decade ago.

Patients and families often ask what attracted me to this sub-specialty in the first place, and like many of my peers it was serendipity, working with an inspirational mentor and possessing a fundamental desire to help patients in genuine need. Invariably, the second question I have been posed is, "How do you cope with all that sadness?", usually followed by the statement, "It must be such a hard job."

I have never particularly thought of my profession as a "job". I guess it is a passion. A passion that has afforded me the rare privilege of accompanying many women (and men) on their unique journey through the challenges of a breast cancer diagnosis. Some journeys are long, too many are short. However, they are all inspirational. I have learnt much from my patients and their families. Extraordinary resilience. The indomitable human spirit. Selflessness and courage in face of dreadful symptoms, the psychological impact of a life-threatening diagnosis and the toxicity of our therapies. As much as possible, I endeavour to put myself in my patients' shoes and more often than not I ponder whether I would cope as well or with such dignity if this was my journey. I doubt I would.

My career has spanned some remarkable therapeutic innovations. Targeted therapies such as herceptin were unavailable when my training began. Our only treatments were surgery, radiation, Tamoxifen and a small coterie of chemotherapy agents. In every aspect of breast cancer management, the last two decades has seen phenomenal change. We have a far better understanding of the molecular pathology of breast cancer, the importance of hereditary susceptibility (such as the BRCA1/2 mutations) and a realisation that each breast cancer has a unique biologic "fingerprint". This now (and even more so in the near future) provides the opportunity to use an individualised or tailored approach to therapy. We are immersed in an era of minimally invasive surgery (such as sentinel node biopsy), better radiotherapy techniques with less side effects, more effective chemotherapy and supportive therapy to enhance tolerability, a number of endocrine agents and "smart" drugs that have been designed to specifically target abnormalities expressed on the surface of breast cancer cells.

My particular interest in breast cancer treatment began in 1996 when I purposefully left Brisbane to study at the Royal Melbourne Hospital, which at the time was leading Australia in the study of using high dose chemotherapy and bone marrow transplantation as a treatment for high risk early breast cancer patients. Having decided that I would like to forge a career in this area, my wife and I moved to Toronto Canada to pursue research as well as start our family. With some irony, the clinical trials I was heavily involved with, when published, proved that bone marrow transplantation was no better than standard chemotherapy. That particular "journey" shuddered to a halt. When I reflect on that period I am quite overwhelmed by not only the "crude" treatment we employed at the time (in comparison with 2018), but the humbly memory of the hundreds of brave women who volunteered to be part of those trials. It has been a relentless common theme over the past 50 years: the preparedness women have had to be involved in clinical trials, often without any guarantee that the trial will help them. It is because of these women our understanding of breast cancer therapy has progressed such a long way.

Undeterred, upon returning to Australia I retained a particular interest in helping care for women who have suffered breast cancer. Despite our advances, it remains a particularly challenging area. Treatments are complex and difficult. The physical, financial and emotional burden of breast cancer is enormous; not only upon the patient but also their families. It requires (if available) teams of highly skilled professionals to help steer the ship. One of the great joys of looking after patients with breast cancer is the ability to interact on a daily basis within a multi-disciplinary team environment. Working with similarly minded, passionate professionals is every bit as inspiring as the women and men affected by this disease.

As I sat and composed this piece, I reflected upon what advice I could offer patients based on a 25-year career in oncology.

We frequently are incapable of explaining why a patient develops breast cancer, or any cancer for that matter. Often it is believed that the entire process begins as a random event. What we can reassure women is that stress, unresolved guilt, childhood trauma and the like have not played any role in the development of their illness. Develop confidence in your treating team and the advice they provide you. If you don't feel that trust, then find another team. Be careful of the internet. Knowledge is empowering... provided it is correct, of course. Your breast cancer is not the same as the next person's. Your treatment may seem the same, but there are often subtle differences that escape chat rooms. Be as critical of internet "cures" as we would expect you to be of more conventional treatments. I've seen the lot: apricot kernels, Japanese mushrooms, shark cartilage, volcanic zeolites, green mussels, coffee enemas, ketogenic diets, microwave therapy, oxygenation, alkalinisation, black cohosh, Gumby Gumby, cannabis oil, etc. If it seems to good to be true, then it probably isn't. Certainly, there is a place for complementary therapies and I personally am quite relaxed about patients pursuing these, and given the potential for interactions with other treatments it is imperative that patients have an open and honest conversation with their nurses and doctors re this.

I am a fan of the concept of "dominating the disease", rather than the converse being true whereby the patient is captive to the illness. Where feasible, patients and families should approach each day positively and try to maintain as much "normality" as possible in their lives. Many of the patients I care for have incurable breast cancer, but I emphasise to them that with modern therapy we can approach cancer as a "chronic disease". Just as patients with diabetes may have periods where their blood sugar is out of control and their medication needs to be adjusted, the same often holds true with cancer treatment.

Finally, I frequently relate to my patients with advanced disease the story of a lady I "inherited" at my first consultant position who had "lived with" metastatic breast cancer for more than 45 years. We usually part with the comment... "So, why shouldn't that be you?"

Qualifications:
MBBS, MMedSc, FRACP

Specialty
Medical Oncologist

Special Interests
Breast Cancer; GIT Cancer; Lung Cancer; Mesothelioma; Urological
Cancer

Phone
07 3737 4500

Fax
07 3737 4877

Address
Icon Cancer Care
Level 1
Sister Edith Centre
Holy Spirit Northside Private Hospital
627 Rode Road
CHERMSIDE QLD 4032

Website
www.iconcancercare.com.au

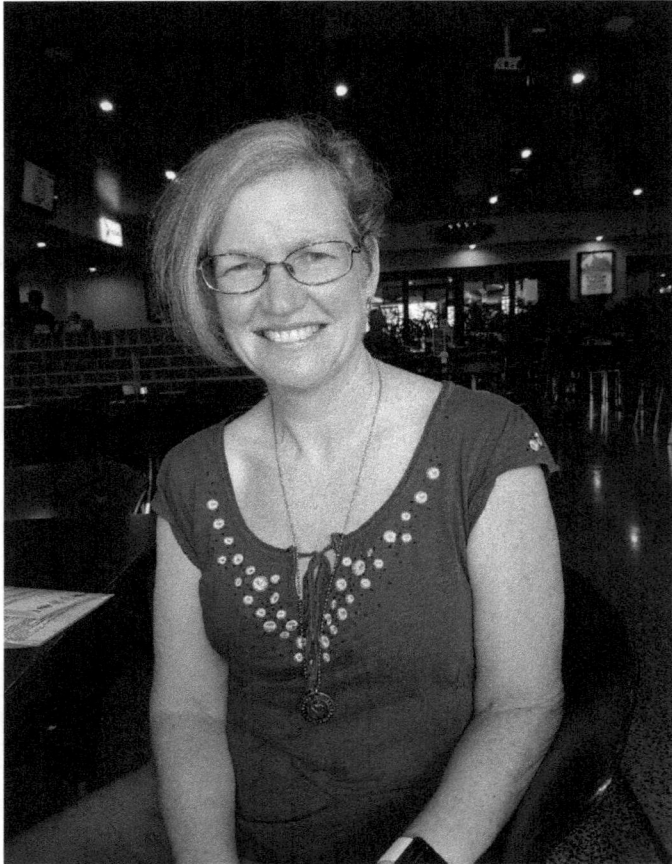

Second Story

By Cheryl Benardos

Cancer – just the thought of it strikes such fear. It seems to so randomly attack, and no-one is immune. As I reflect on how cancer has affected my life, I realise that no less than 10 people I know have battled breast cancer (probably more), some still with us and some not. Not to mention those diagnosed with other forms of cancer, including my own darling Mum who died of lung cancer in 2007.

One of my aunts was barely 40 years old when she passed away – far too young to die. I remember her funeral clearly. I had only been to one or two funerals before that, and the depth of emotion around me that day was very intense. I remember the grief-stricken face of my grandmother and thinking that it seems so wrong to outlive your child.

Another beloved aunty was diagnosed with breast cancer in one breast, and after surviving that she was diagnosed with a different form of breast cancer in the other breast. Thankfully, she survived that too, although she has since passed away and I miss her dearly. She always had such a positive outlook and I remember her saying to me, "Shit happens. You just have to get on with life."

I remember attending a funeral for a young mum whose children attended the school I work at. She was only in her early 30's. It was a beautiful service celebrating her life. Looking at her children that day was heartbreaking. Tears streamed down my face as I felt their loss – all the milestones that their mum wouldn't be there for. Their lives were forever changed.

One dear friend of mine has been through hell and back, and thankfully she is still with us. After surgery and chemotherapy, she then faced a major operation for breast reconstruction. I can see that although this time she has triumphed, cancer still continues to be her silent companion. The dread of each check-up followed by relief with the all clear. Trying to keep life stress free for fear of retriggering the cancer.

Cancer has already had such a devastating impact on my life. How do you face the reality of the disease and yet stay positive? This has often plagued me, as a good mental attitude is so important, yet it is no good being in denial – such a fine line to tread.

I have witnessed great courage in the face of this disease. The physical and emotional battles that are fought. My perspective comes from that of a loved one. It is so hard to watch someone I care about suffering. I feel such a sense of helplessness. My mum never talked to me about dying. I think she was worried that I would get too upset. Sometimes I wish we had talked about it, because at times it felt like it was the elephant in the room.

Then there is the grief. Crying a river of tears. The finality of loss. Wishes unfulfilled. Being cheated by time. The void that can't be filled.

It is funny how little things can strike you when you least expect it. Whenever I see a Mother's Day card or a Mum birthday card and realise I never will buy one again I am filled with immense sadness. But the things I miss the most about Mum are our conversations, and being able to hug her.

Each time I have a mammogram there is a tiny seed of anxiety – what if?? – and a breath of relief with the all clear. And then I remind myself that each day I am here is a blessing – make the most of it!!!

Cheryl Bernados is 51 years old with 3 daughters living in Brisbane. She loves her job working as a prep teacher aide and has been with Education Queensland for the past 18 years. She has struggled with depression since losing her mum to cancer in 2007. She says she feels very honoured to have been asked to contribute to this book.

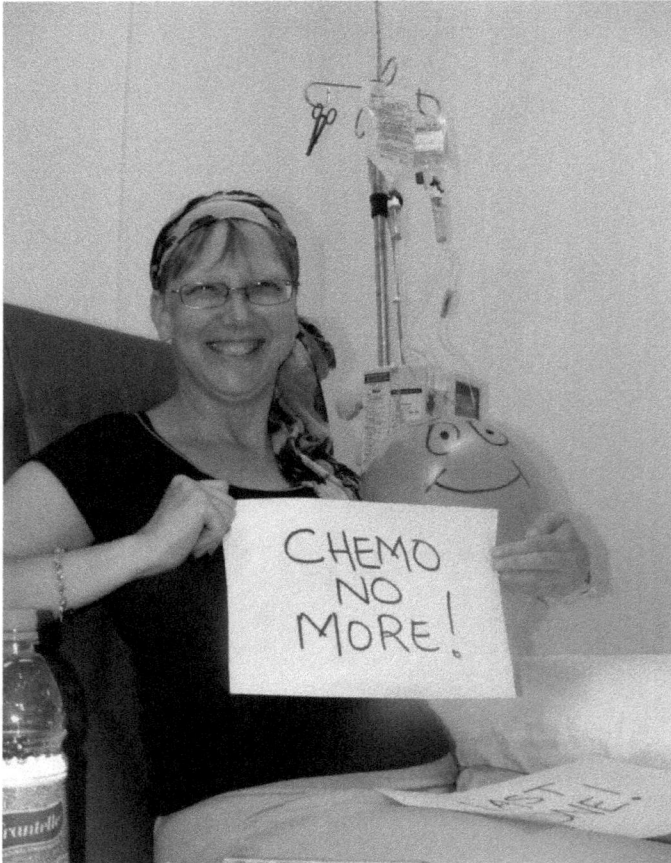

Third Story

By Andy Kahle

They say bad luck comes in 3s, if you believe in all that stuff. And while I'm not a superstitious person, I reckon it's probably true. How do I know?

Well, back in 2009 my hubby and I decided that we were over playing with other people's drag racing cars, and it was time to bite the bullet and get one of our own. This didn't take too long to sort out, as a good friend of ours, Simon, just happened to have the perfect car sitting on the hoist in his workshop. A Granny Smith green, 1969, 2 door LC Torana with a small block Chev engine.

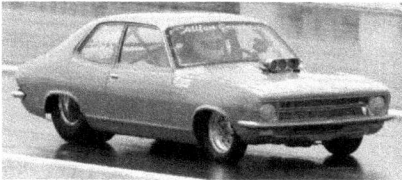

It was just meant to be. Both of us are 1969 babies, and my very first car was an LC Torana.

So, I handed the man some money and we all got to work in his workshop making modifications to the car and training me how to drive it.

You would think if you know how to drive a car, you'd know how to drive a drag car, wouldn't you? But no. It's actually quite different. Simon has been drag racing for what seems like forever, so it was the obvious choice that he not only guide Mick through maintaining a drag racing engine, but also teach and mentor me in the art of driving.

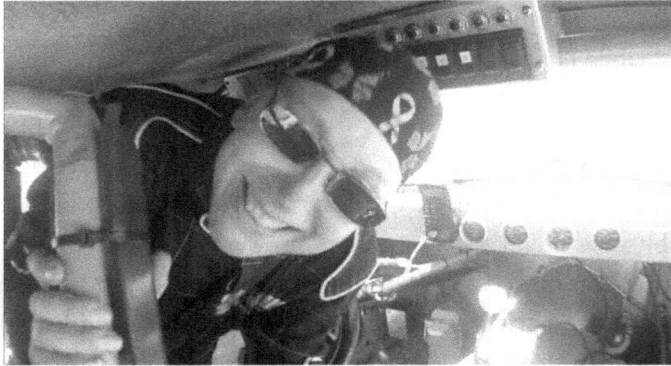

So arrives the day before my first day on track. The car is ready, and apparently so am I. I didn't feel ready. I was so nervous that I was sure I would make a total fool of myself in front of everyone.

"OK, so let's just do some practise in my car park," Simon suggested. He's not talking actual speed racing, just doing a burnout and launching the car, since at this point I had only done it in pretend, not with the actual engine running.

So, we clean out the car park of anything I might hit like bins, other cars, random feral cats etc., opened up the gates just in case I forget to brake, and put some witches hats out on the road. Luckily, it's a very quiet street, and I won't tell you exactly where because I'm sure there were some legal issues with what we were doing.

So, I suit up in all my gear, get strapped into the driver's seat and the boys push the car all the way back to the far end of the car park. Mick puts a little water down to help with the burnout process, and Simon sets up a pretend start line. It's great. I practise doing the burnout, which after a couple of goes didn't seem too difficult all. I'm actually starting to feel much less nervous about hitting the track tomorrow.

Time to practise the launch sequence. Now, this is a little more complicated; there's buttons to push and then let go at the same time as you put your foot to floor, and switches to throw and tacho to watch and the lights to watch and the temperature gauge to watch and ... what's all that smoke coming out of the transmission? and it stinks...

Why are Simon and Mick waving their arms about... OH... shut it down... OK.

So apparently it was the most melted convertor that Simon had ever seen before in his life. And he's a converter specialist. Apparently, you're not supposed to sit on the trans brake for an entire minute with the engine at high revs ... about 3 seconds is the maximum or everything melts and the transmission fluid starts to burn and smoke. Oops.

It's going to be a long night if we still want to get out on track tomorrow. So, as bad as I feel about screwing up, I pitch in and help remove the transmission from the car and pull out the converter. I rush the transmission over to Mr D around the corner, who promises to drop everything and freshen it up right away. And Simon sends Mick and me home to relax with the promise that he will work all night to get it all back together again. I'm amazed that these people would do this for me, but over the years I've found out that this is just what the drag racing family does.

So that was one... but at this point who is counting. You don't count when you only have one.

Once home, I'm the first to jump in the shower to remove all that grease and grime, while Mick feeds the dogs. Then I start sorting out a late dinner while Mick goes for his shower.

"Andy." ... "Andy."

There's no urgency in the call, so I figure he's just run out of soap or something.

I pop my head through the bathroom doorway only to see my strapping 6ft man standing just out of the running water, looking whiter than the bathroom tiles holding his arm up with blood running down his side and down the drain.

"I think I need an ambulance," he said, ever so calmly. He had slipped in the shower and impaled his arm on the tap, severing muscle and tendon and making quite a mess of himself.

So, again, I'm apologising to Simon and Mr D for messing them about. After all, the doctors are looking at sending Mick in for micro surgery tomorrow instead of Mick sending me out on the race track for the first time.

So that was two. And this is the point where you do become a little wary as you're waiting for that other shoe to drop.

Mick's arm was well on the mend and while the drag racing season was starting to wrap up, Simon, Mick and I had worked out that we should be able to sneak in a couple of testing days at the track before winter sets in.

Well, that was what we thought, until I found a lump in my breast.

On the 30th of March 2010, my GP confirmed that bad luck comes in 3s. I had breast cancer. And a particularly aggressive one at that. There would be no drag racing this season or indeed the next season, as I was about to have the fight of my life on my hands.

Once again, I found myself apologising to Simon and Mr D.

Drag racing was going to have to take a back seat. But it was just a delay. I knew it would just be a matter of time. I pasted photos of my drag car in the front of my medical diary and showed anyone who showed the slightest interest. Nurses, doctors, other patients, the tea lady, even the young girl who came in to mop the floor in my hospital room knew my goal. And they would all smile encouragingly, probably thinking I was a nutter, but at least they didn't say so out loud.

Late at night, laying in the hospital bed, IV's hanging out my arm, oxygen mask strapped on, and for some reason not being able to sleep, I'd look at those photos.

I'll kick this. I will drive you, little green Torana. And not just in someone's car park.

On days when I didn't feel too sick, Mick would take me to Simon's workshop, and while he helped work on Simon's own drag car, I'd sit in mine, willing myself to be well enough to finally get on track and race.

The boys even dragged me down to the track, just to watch. And the smell and atmosphere only made the need to kick this stupid cancer and drive even stronger.

Finally, it was time. I'd won. No more drugs, no more radiation, no more surgery. I'd done it. With the support all around me and a huge goal set in my head that I needed to achieve, I'd managed to kick cancer to the curb.

So, the question on everyone's lips is... did I finally get to drive?

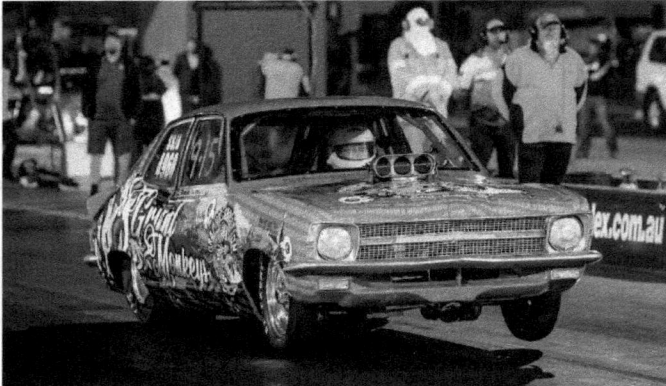

Hell Yeah!

On the 29th of October 2011, my post chemo hair still short and very curly, surrounded by some amazing friends and an immensely proud hubby, I stood up on stage to accept the runner up trophy for my very first drag race.

And I haven't look back since. I now race every chance I get and I share my passion with anyone who will listen. We all have to have a dream to focus on when times are tough, but how many can actually say they went out and achieved it?

Face your fears and live your dreams!!

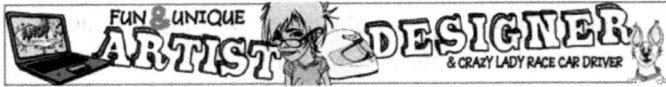

FUN & UNIQUE ARTIST DESIGNER & CRAZY LADY RACE CAR DRIVER

Andy Kahle (or Andrea when she's in trouble) is a graphic designer, artist, wife, sister, friend, daughter, small business owner, and motorsport enthusiast, in no particular order. She was born in Victoria but grew up in a small Pilbara town in North Western Australia, and now lives with her husband of 27 years in Perth, Western Australia. Shortly after turning 40, with no history of cancer in her family and no history of ill health in her own life, she was diagnosed with breast cancer. Now, after being clear for 7 years, she volunteers for a local breast cancer charity to help others who don't have the support that she was lucky enough to have through treatment.

Andy Kahle
andy@andyk.com.au
Ph: 0437312394

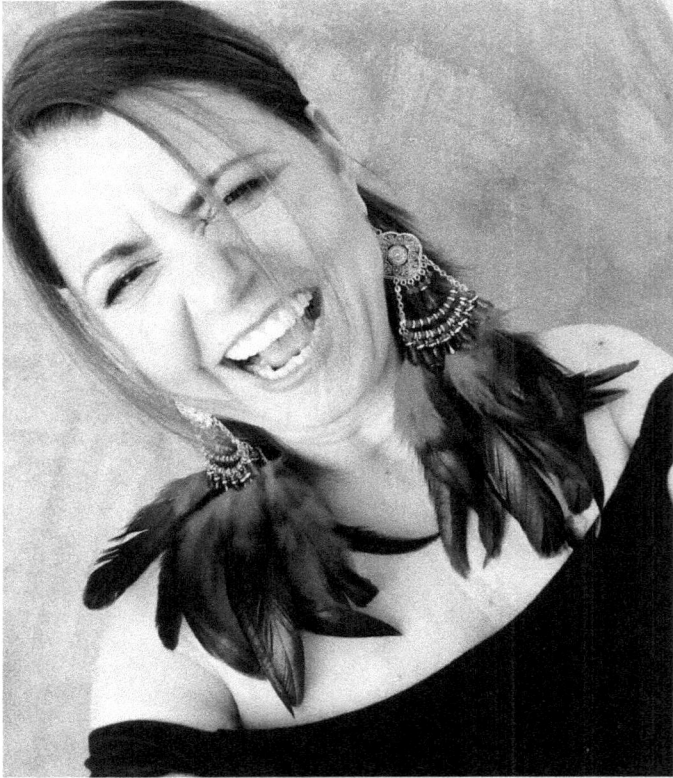

Fourth Story

by Kassandra Behrendt

It's 2007 and I'm in a good place. My daughter is five years old. I only have one child, Samara, because I just kept miscarrying, and earlier that year I'd had a miscarriage and the baby was 11 weeks old. We'd already heard the heartbeat, but then when we went back for the regular ultrasound they couldn't find a heartbeat and they found that the baby was dead, so I had to go into hospital and have it removed.

That was early part of 2007 and we kept chugging along and things are good. Samara is five and she's a brilliant child, and we decide not to try for another.

I was working on my jewellery design business, doing a lot of party planning at that time and it was quite successful. It was all word of mouth and this was before the GFC, so people were just spending money and it was so easy to sell. People would invite me into their homes and I had set up a party plan structure, but it was just me and nobody else was working for me.

Come November 2007, however, and I decided that I had a health list. I decided I'm just going to tick everything off. I was feeling fantastic. I'd lost weight. I just felt fabulous and I thought I'll just tick the breast cancer thing off the list and go and get a mammogram, because my mother died of breast cancer, and I thought, 'Nah, that wouldn't happen to me.'

So, I went to have a mammogram and a week later they phoned me on a Friday to say, "You need to come back in for more tests." So, I went in on Monday with my husband Greg as my support and they said, "We just need to do some biopsies." So, they take cells out of my breast and say, "Come back tomorrow and we'll let you know what the results are." I didn't feel anything and definitely didn't feel there was a lump.

So, they took cells out of my breast and then I went back the next day without Greg thinking it's nothing to worry about, and they proceeded to tell me the different stages of breast cancer. One was when they just find a little lump in the breast that they can surgically remove. Two is a little bit bigger and the breasts might have to be removed. Three is when it's moved outside the breast and outside of the lymph nodes. And so, they tell me that three is where I am.

Because I was not expecting this outcome, I was going to go shopping afterwards as a type of reward. Instead, I went into the car and I called Greg and I said, "Are you alone?" He goes, "No, just hold on a minute". He's always running meetings. I said, "It's cancer, and it's spread." There was no way to say it nicely. Then I asked him to come home.

I cried all the way home. I got home and then Greg came in, and he started crying so I had to be the strong one because Greg is usually strong, but sometimes he's not. And we swap, like when the baby had to be removed, I cried and cried and then when he started crying I stopped and soothed him. I thought I was going to die, that it was just a matter of time.

Before the surgery we were very practical. We got a lawyer, so Greg could have Power of Attorney in case I die on the operating table. We made sure everything was in his name so that everything could be taken care of. And we cried.

Then came the surgery and the surgeon had to take more than she initially thought. She wanted to do a lumpectomy, but I said, "No, just remove the whole thing." You just don't know what's going on. "But," I added, "Do not touch my tattoo. You cut around my tattoo." When I woke up I was flat on one side and I thought, 'alright then, what now?'.

It was lucky we removed the whole breast, because it had spread everywhere. It was like a fire cancer, no lumps, nobody would ever have felt it. It was only the mammogram that picked up a little bit of shading. She sent me home and said, "I'll call you".

So, I went home, and she called me back to say, "We have to do more surgery to remove more lymph nodes because it has spread beyond what we removed." So, they cut out a bit more than they need to make sure that they've got all the cancer. Then I went back to find out it had spread beyond those lymph nodes.

Greg and I are just walking around like ghosts and we're trying to be normal. He took some time off work, but we kept what was happening mostly to ourselves and didn't tell everybody.

We were just walking around like ghosts doing regular things until it was my birthday on the 17th of December. I'd been crying all morning and Greg said, "Why don't we go shopping?" Because if you want to cheer me up, you just take me shopping. He took me to my favourite shops wanting to know, "What do you think of this?" and "What do you think of that?" But my heart just wasn't in it.

What's the point of buying pretty things if you are going to be dying? Then I got a phone call from my surgeon and she said, "It's clear, you're fine". So, Greg went and bought me a dress, and I still have that dress. I called some close friends as soon as we got home and said, "Party at my place, it's all clear". And so, they all came.

Then it was back to the practical stuff like having to go and have all my wisdom teeth removed before chemotherapy. Something about infection and trying to avoid it during chemo.

My God, it was awful. The dentist had his knees on either side of me on the chair and the nurse was holding me down. What an awful experience.

It was a difficult time because my oncologist thought we should do chemo every second week to get it done in three months instead of every three or four weeks over a longer period of time. I had to get a porta Cath connected to my major vein so that they could put the chemotherapy through there, so I go in to do that and he couldn't find a vein to give me general anaesthetic. He cut me open without general anaesthetic and put the porta Cath in and then he gave me the general. It was the worst experience of my life. It was awful. They didn't even give me a local to do that.

Anyway, I got that done and then I started chemotherapy and I started losing my hair. It just kept falling out in chunks, and we had to tell Samara that Mummy's sick and she's going to lose her hair. My hair was way down my back. It was beautiful, long and blonde, and it was traumatic as my hands were going through my hair and all these big chunks were coming out.

Samara just loved playing with my hair, and we would give her some masking tape and she would put it on my hand and peel it off, like giving me a wax; and hair would come off doing that. She would do that every day until all my hair came out, and she loved it. And then she painted my head and my face in rainbow colours.

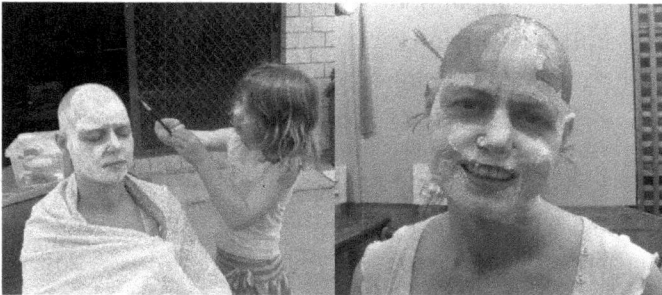

We tried to make it a game for her, but she knew something was going on. Children sense these things. Then her wonderful little girlfriend's mother went into hospital for standard surgery and died. And so, every time I went into hospital for Chemo, Samira would cling on to my leg, not wanting to let me go thinking I wasn't going to come home.

This was just too much. Anyway. So, I had the breast removed, I had chemotherapy, I had radiation, I had hormonal therapy, and then a year later they took the porta Cath out because my treatment was done.

I couldn't get a reconstruction, so I had one breast and I was wearing a bra with a prosthetic thing which made it look ok when I was wearing clothes, but it would constantly get itchy because it was summer.

When I was finally able to have a reconstruction, it didn't work. When you put a foreign object in your body and the body creates a capsule around it, it thinks it's an infection. It's fun. And that's normal. But this one became like a rock and I had to go back in and put another one in, and that one was okay. But the plastic surgeon did such a horrible job. I mean, I've seen other women who've had breast reconstruction. They had one noodle scar across the top and that's it.

After all that, I had to go back every month to get the other breast examined to make sure that the cancer hadn't spread to that breast because that's standard when you've got breast cancer in one. And they wouldn't just do an ultrasound, they would do biopsies, and this breast was constantly bruised, and it was getting smaller and smaller. I ended up with two breasts of different sizes, different textures.

I then had the procedure where they take the muscle from the back around the front, but it's still connected to the blood banks. Then they'll put an extra implant in as well. It's not ideal and I have to go to the physio and she has to do special things.

Anyway, after all this, I was well again, and everybody went their separate ways. But I became really depressed, even became suicidal. I felt that I was a burden to everybody, to my family. I now understand people who are depressed and suicidal because you reach that point where you think that nobody would miss you. You think that you're so worthless and such a waste of space, you need to kill yourself so that others can get on with their lives, and that's the space that I was.

In hindsight now, I think, 'How could I've left my five-year-old baby alone?' We had never been apart ever since she was born. I didn't go to work. We were always together. She adored me, and my husband adored me too. I had read statistics during that time where I think up to 85 percent of husbands left their wives once they were diagnosed with breast cancer.

I said that to Greg and he said, "No, I'll never leave you." He said, "They can cut off your arms, they can cut off your legs, as long as it's you, I will always be with you. Of course I will still love you."

Still, I was angry all the time. I was yelling for no reason. I was yelling at Greg. I was unhappy. So angry, constantly angry. I felt worthless and just left out and it was totally unreasonable. But you're not very reasonable in that state.

I was an abused child and I witnessed a lot of the abuse my mother received. He would hit her in front of me and he would then bash me up and we couldn't have any friends or have anybody over. So, I grew up very withdrawn and sad and feeling worthless.

When I met Greg, he made me feel so loved. I felt cherished. I felt safe. It was just fantastic. Yet here I was, depressed and suicidal.

I had a history of being suicidal, and all of that came back. I began asking, 'Why me?' My breasts were my best feature, and so was my hair. I used to walk around without a bra, even after breastfeeding, as my breasts were still beautiful, and it was attached to my femininity. I had to go for a whole year with one breast on one side, and this ugly scar.

Then to have a reconstruction that didn't work and then to have another reconstruction. Then have the other one removed, and no nipples. My nipples were my best asset, especially during sex, but let's not go there.

It's like, I can't feel anything, but I have to be careful what I wear. If I wear a strapless something it has to be really tight. Otherwise it'll fall down, and I won't feel it. It actually happened to me once.

This is when a very good friend was trying to reach me. Greg couldn't reach me. He doesn't understand how people can get depressed. He just doesn't, he just doesn't understand, so I didn't tell him and especially didn't tell him that I was suicidal, but I did tell my best friend because she could read me. You know how girls can read each other, and she knew I was not in a good place. She said, "You have to go and talk to somebody."

So, I finally reached a point where I thought, 'Either fucking kill yourself or get some help.' So that was a real bottom. I was constantly yelling at my daughter and then I felt like shit because I was yelling at her, so I went and saw a psychologist. It took me a couple of goes, but I found this one woman who really is just like a girlfriend. We just connected, and I knew that she could feel, that she had empathy. She wasn't just clinical. She suggested I start some antidepressants to help clear my head I agreed. I tried three different ones before I found the one that worked, but it was like I woke up and there was this cloud lifted off my brain and everything was clear.

So much has happened in my life since then, but I want to leave you with this:

Get regular mammograms so that you don't get breast cancer.

Be honest with the people that love you. You can't do this on your own. I think people need to self-love themselves enough to know that the people that love them need to be involved in the experience and the journey and that you are not alone.

I realised that I am resilient. Bloody resilient. I cannot believe how many times I've been knocked down and just picked myself up again. Strong as fuck. Balance.

Honestly, I look back and I often think about those days and I think I did okay, but now, talking to you now, I've actually sat down and actually spent time thinking about, and I think, 'Shit, that was fucking awful.' It *was* awful. But I am here, and I have survived. So can you.

Pagoni: www.pagoni.com
Email: Kassandra@pagoni.com
Ph: 0411 434 666

In 1972, eight-year-old Kassandra and her family boarded the ship 'Patris' in Greece, to begin the long journey to Australia. Along with thousands of other young Greek children, she started school, learning English and how to fit into to her new home.

Despite a traumatic childhood, she threw herself into her corporate career after attending secretarial studies at TAFE. But in her heart, Kassandra is a creative spirit, and she started designing jewellery. What started as a hobby grew into a profitable and fulfilling business. A self-taught jewellery designer, she taps into her Greek heritage with her bold and feminine designs. Her business grew from designing a few pieces here and there to match her flamboyant and elegant outfits to women requesting pieces for themselves.

Today, Kassandra's pieces are in demand, appearing on covers of magazines and sought after by high profile and powerful women. But her true passion lies in giving back ... coupled with her incredible design skills, she volunteers for several not-for-profit organisations. As a survivor of childhood abuse and breast cancer, those organisations are close to her heart. She is driven to give back, often donating her pieces to charities and groups to help them raise much needed funds. Her generosity is only matched by her humility.

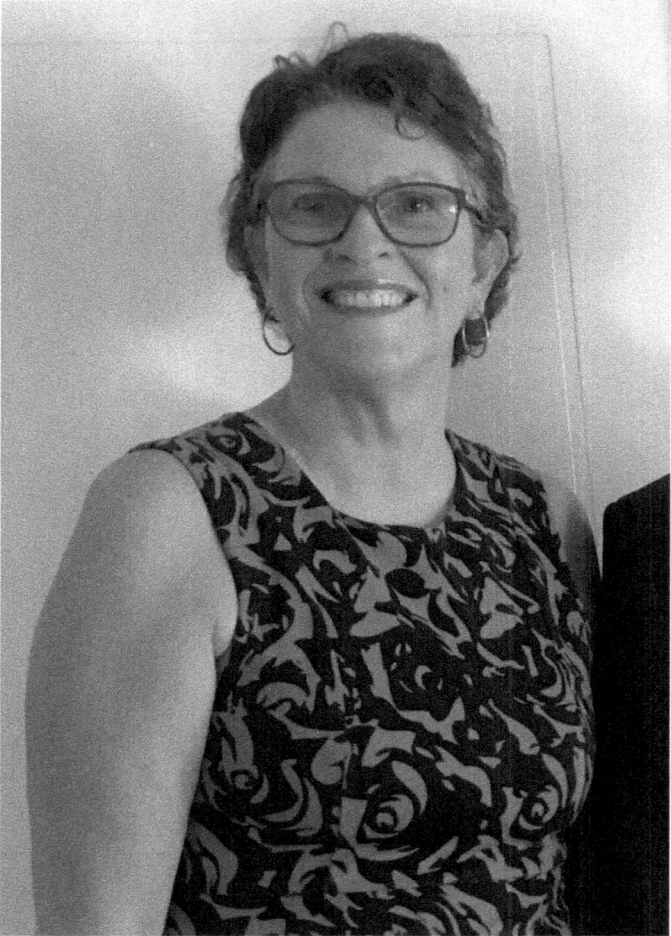

Fifth Story

By Helen Roche

There is no good place to be when you are first told you have cancer. For me, it was driving home from work to pick up my children from school. I received a phone call from the radiologist and she asked me if I was sitting somewhere comfortably. I was on Brisbane's inner-city bypass. I couldn't stop and I had to get my kids. I took a deep breath and asked her to just tell me. Time waits for no Cancer.

She advised me that I had a small breast cancer. There was that word that none of us want to hear in the same sentence as our name. I felt myself go clammy. I listened as she explained everything, and then I drove and cried. Cancer happens to other people. My kids are still young, I love my husband and my life. Why me?

In January 2014, just over 12 months after I had celebrated my 50th birthday in Italy with close friends in a joy filled, decadent, sumptuous week of partying, I felt a small lump in my left breast. I wasn't overly concerned as I knew that I had dense breasts and had previously felt lumps that turned out to be fibroadenomas and completely harmless.

Nevertheless, always one to err on the side of caution, I took myself off to my lovely GP for an examination. She gave me a thorough examination, agreed with me that it was probably nothing to be worried about, but suggested I go and have a mammogram and ultrasound just to be on the safe side. I have been having regular checks by BreastScreen Queensland since I was 45, and results have always shown no areas of concern.

I made an appointment and arrived at Diagnostic Imaging for Women on 9th February 2015. I was given a mammogram and ultra sound and sent to the waiting room where I expected to be told that everything was fine and to get dressed and go back to my life. After a short wait, I was asked to come back into the ultrasound room where I was met by two radiologists. They explained to me that whilst the lump I had felt in my left breast appeared to be harmless, there was in fact a slight anomaly in my right breast, and they would like to do a fine needle aspiration biopsy to be sent off to pathology.

Of course, I agreed. I was given a local anaesthetic in my breasts (they decided to take a sample of the lump in the left breast as well) and a needle was inserted, and a small amount of tissue taken. This was relatively painless. I went home to wait for the results, still feeling confident that all would be well.

On Monday I received a phone call from the head radiologist at DIW. She told me that the pathologists needed a further sample from my right breast to be able to completely rule out any issues. My heart started to beat a little faster at this point, but the C word had not been mentioned, so I was happy to stay in my safe place for now. I was asked to come back for a Stereotactic biopsy.

I was advised that this procedure would be more invasive, but also more accurate. This type of biopsy uses mammograms to pinpoint the location of suspicious areas within the breast. For this procedure, I had to lie face-down on a padded biopsy table with my right breast positioned in a hole in the table. It was quite uncomfortable, and I could not move or see anything except the wall for about 45 minutes.

The table was raised several feet, and the equipment used by the radiologist was positioned beneath the table. My breast was firmly compressed between two plates while mammograms were taken to show the radiologist the exact location of the area for biopsy.

The radiologist made a small incision, about 6 millimetres, into my breast. She then inserted a needle and removed several samples of tissue. Even as I write this now, three years after the procedure, I am in tears. I felt so vulnerable, uncertain and very scared even though the nurse and radiologist were very kind.

Three days later I received THAT phone call as I was driving.

My type of breast cancer is called Invasive Lobular Carcinoma and it begins in the milk-producing glands (lobules) of the breast. Invasive cancer means the cancer cells have broken out of the lobule where they began and have the potential to spread to the lymph nodes and other areas of the body. I would require surgery, radiation and perhaps chemotherapy. The prognosis was good as it was very early days.

After that phone call, things moved very quickly, just as time seemed to stand still. I told my husband, who was on the bus at the time, but I just had to tell somebody. I told my family, but not my kids. I needed more information before I did that. I went to my GP, got a referral to a surgeon, had the process explained to me, and was booked in to have surgery within a week of diagnosis. I am very grateful that we are in a position to have private health cover. I am also very grateful to the McGrath Foundation and all Breast Cancer Foundations that have raised money and awareness. I received a lot of information, soft bras for post-surgery and was assigned a Breast Care Nurse, Natasha, who was a godsend in guiding me through the process of what was happening to me.

The day before surgery, I had a small amount of radioactive material injected into my right breast so the surgeon could identify the sentinel node/s. These are the lymph nodes that the breast drains to first. They are the first lymph nodes to which cancer cells are most likely to spread from a primary breast tumour. My sentinel nodes were identified under my arm and near my breast bone.

The next morning at 6 o'clock on the 6th March 2015, I arrived at the hospital with my husband. I was very emotional and scared. I couldn't stop crying or shaking. I will be eternally grateful to Natasha who held my hand. As ILC is not visible to the naked eye, I had to have a wire guide inserted so that the surgeon would know where to cut. This was done in a similar manor to the stereotactic biopsy. I was then taken to surgery crying and shaking in a hospital gown with wires sticking out of my breasts.

I woke up with the feeling that somebody was sitting on my chest and I couldn't breathe. I was panicking. Why couldn't I breathe, it hurt so much. My surgeon was there in recovery, which in my fog I thought was strange. He explained to me that while they were trying to remove the sentinel node in my chest, my lung had been punctured. That was why I felt like I couldn't breathe. Apart from that, he said all went well. It was now just a matter of waiting for a few days to see if they got it all. A few days? What could be easier?

I remained in hospital for two more days. The pain was bad, but the drugs they gave me to ease it made me sick. It was a matter of deciding which was the lesser of two evils. I put up with the pain.

Being told that I had cancer was bad, but the four days of waiting for the results were worse. My mind went to all the terrible places – I feared that the cancer was everywhere, I was going to die, I would need another operation, I would lose my breasts, and on and on it went. By Wednesday, I couldn't sleep, and I felt like I was having a panic attack. Just when I thought I couldn't last another minute, the surgeon rang me. They had got it all. I sat on the lounge and cried and cried. You can see there is a theme here, can't you?

And so, six weeks of radiation, no chemotherapy, ten years of taking tamoxifen and anastrozole that threw me into menopause, gave me hot flushes and arthritis, and I'm back. I'm Helen again. But is it really that easy? No!! There comes a point where everyone who has had a life-threatening disease or experience must face it. The story I told myself for many months was that it was only a little cancer, they got it all, I was never going to die, I didn't need chemotherapy so there were people a lot worse off than me. I just went back to my life and tried to pretend that everything was the same. It wasn't. It never will be!

We need to be gentle with ourselves. We need to grieve for the loss, whether it is one breast, two or just the scars left from surgery and radiation. Everybody's journey is their own and they are all valid. Don't compare yourself to somebody else who has had cancer. Take time to heal. Ask for help and talk about how you feel. I am blessed to have a wonderful husband and family who supported me through my journey which continues to this day. Every year as I sit in the waiting room for the results of my mammogram and ultrasound, I relive that first time three years ago and hold my breath until they tell me all is well.

You can reach Helen at:
helen_roche@hotmail.com

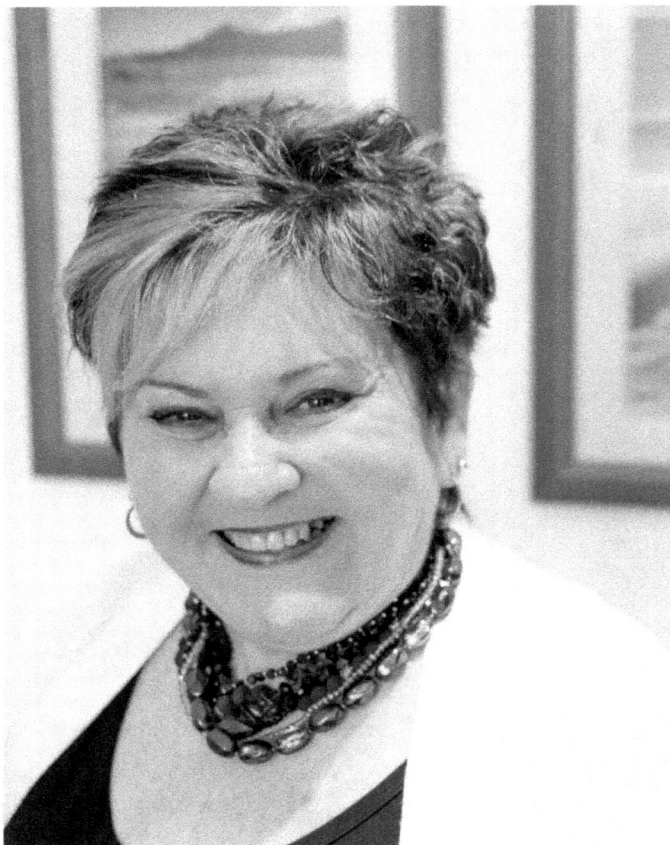

Sixth Story

By Pat Armitstead

Threads of life – holding on and letting go.

> *"In Greek mythology,*
> *Gaia was the mother goddess*
> *who presided over the earth.*
> *In my business, Joyology,*
> *Gaia was the friend goddess*
> *who presided over my soul."*
> *- Pat Armitstead*

We'd been distant friends for many years, meeting infrequently. That is, until the day of her first diagnosis. It was then a mutual friend who sought me out and quietly said, "Pat, I think you should meet and talk with Gaia about your work". And so I did, and on that day at the close of our conversation, she politely declined the experience I offered, saying, "Pat, I am just going to heal this without any outside intervention".

I remember we were standing by the fridge as she put away some organic produce.

And so it was that she defied medical advice and other interventions, ate about 85% organically and created a meditation where she envisaged a field of flowers moving ever so gently in the breeze... inside her cancerous breast! In less than 12 months, there was no sign of cancer in her breast!

Yes, that meditation was her only practice.

We met increasingly over the ensuing 5 years, enjoying the sunshine, the sharing of tales from our lives, gentle repartee and our evolving consciousness. She wrote her book *Genitals, Love and Other Bits and Pieces* (yes, it's as good as it sounds!) and enjoyed the fruits of that labour. I had further developed my Good Grief program, where I continued to cast people with ailments or moving though grief and loss, capturing and releasing stuck emotions and making meaning and beauty with the resultant cast sculptures.

What Gaia would not have known at that point is that, in the lead up to developing the Good Grief program, I had worked with four Jungian Psychotherapists for a 12-month period. We had met monthly, sharing current personal issues and challenges, exploring and sharing myths, legends, fairy-tales, symbolism, colour and crystals to make art and meaning of our current "ailments". We used a casting process popularized by Christiane Corbat before her passing in 2006. http://www.christianecorbat.com/

This experience became the foundation of my Good Grief program.

Gaia's phone call at the end of that 5th year took me by surprise. She said, "I think I would like to do what you suggested years ago. The breast cancer has returned in my other breast. Can you come and tell me more?" We talked at length, enjoying another level of intimacy, and she shared the cancer's return and revealed that she also had Parkinson's Disease, the tremors noticeable by now, and had never been able to heal or slow its progress.

She said to me on that day, "I could heal this cancer again, but I don't want to die of Parkinson's, and for that reason I am going to surrender to the cancer."

Over the next 12 months she stepped out on a journey revisiting past relationships and healing every little wound there was in her association with others. Part of that was spent with both of us going on retreat (or perhaps we should call it a "forward") to become one with nature and to make art and meaning of this unfolding 12-month period. A chance encounter at a water cooler at Auckland Hospital had Gaia connect with the owner of a magical property purpose built to be a sanctuary for healing. We spent four days there, just being with the wonderful connections with nature.

The first night a dragonfly arrived and sat high on her mosquito net. The dragonfly, in almost every part of the world, symbolizes change, and change in the perspective of self-realization; the kind of change that has its source in mental and emotional maturity and the understanding of the deeper meaning of life. The traditional association of dragonflies with water also gives rise to the meaning to this amazing insect. The dragonfly's scurrying flight across water represents an act of going beyond what's on the surface and looking into the deeper implications and aspects of life. This affirmed and further guided our conversations and became a tangible piece of the art with us attaching a dragonfly.

We spent 4 days in this retreat where every tree was a different species, and every moss on every tree bore no likeness to the other! If ever there was a garden that fairies lived in, it was here. The hours just unfolded, night and day unfolded and we followed our intuition, preparing the canvas and discussing what was to be captured. Layer upon layer was painted on the canvas, cementing our intentions and honouring the canvas as the place to hold this final form. The last 24 hours we were ready to cast, and we began this intimate capture of what was sitting in the left torso and face and what was to be held by the right hand. Once the cast was touch dry, we created a ceremony and ritual around it, blessing what had just unfolded and making prayer for what we wanted it to hold.

I remember Gaia exclaiming about her droopy boobs, which caught me a little off guard but showed me how we experience attachment to our younger form, which we perceive to be more beautiful! Casting always reveals any area the body is out of alignment, and so it was for Gaia too. Her left shoulder was lower than the right, but rather than show that she chose to have the shoulder straight, even though it then meant her neck and face would be slightly angled, as you will see in the images.

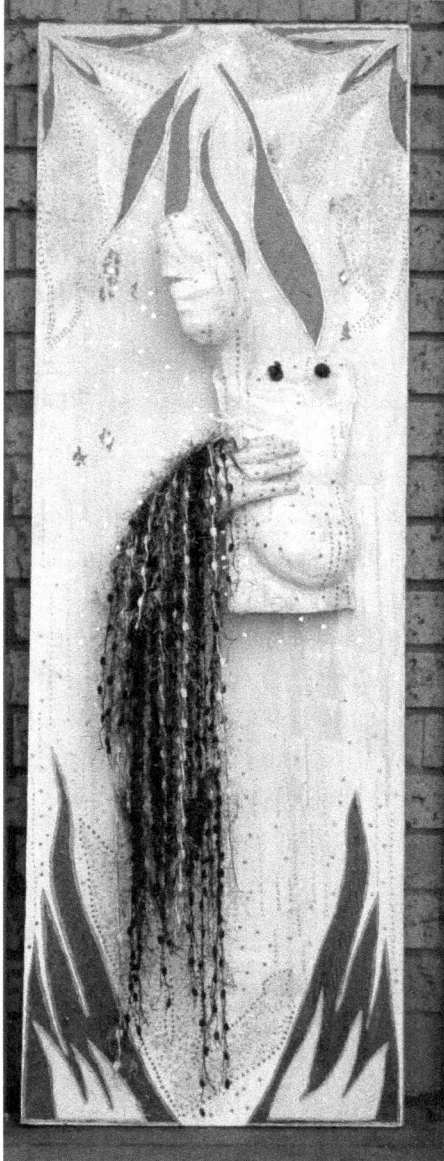

Her right hand was cast over her heart, and on completion, holds the threads of life. The knots in the wool symbolised all the components of her life, the synchronous moments and the journey of the last 12 months, revisiting every conversation and cleaning up the past. The small gold stars, hard to see in a photo, reflect the fairy garden we worked in. And so, the visual was completed well before her passing and she had it in her home until the imminent approach of her demise, when she was hospitalized.

Have you ever wanted to have that one last conversation with somebody, but they passed before you could? Or, perhaps you are afraid you will pass before you can create this conversation? Well, imagine the reverse of that, and the person who had died returning to have that last conversation with you! Along with the piece of art "Threads of Life" displayed on the day, Gaia had us play her recorded final conversation, addressed to family and friends. To unexpectedly hear her voice, her dulcet tones and endearing humour, was amusing, hugely poignant and significant! For Gaia, this was the final catharsis, the art and the journey to clean up the past being the first stage, and this the final closing piece.

(The entire audio can be heard at: https://www.youtube.com/watch?v=UYUQ903gh68)

"Hello to you... you didn't really think I would leave without some final words to you, did you? Heck... no interruptions... one final bit of wisdom... hmm... ego, Gaia, ego. One final sharing while still able to do so. However, as you are listening to me one last time, it means that I've dipped my paddle into the current as I float along the never-ending stream of continuous life. Row, row, row your boat… gently down the stream…

I didn't have to pack a bag, I didn't even have to take my body with me. And, in fact, I didn't even choose to take any of my baggage with me.

No bag. No body. No Baggage.

Just free to be me. So, did I leave with any regrets? I always thought I'd leave with regrets. Things I had done, I wished I had not done. Things I hadn't done, that I wished I had. But now, I am poised… ready to paddle into part of the stream of life we call death. Experienced often, but seldom remembered. And I realised I will be leaving without one single regret to slow me down.

All those "if only"s …. "shoulds" … "coulds" … "why did I"s… times I could have tried harder, but didn't. All those times comparing myself to others and found myself failing. All those times I'd decided I was superior… or inferior to someone else. The numerous stories I'd told myself and others that just weren't true. When I would have given anything to have changed the decision I'd made and the actions that went with that decision. In other words, to have never done a certain deed or action toward someone else, that having done so I regretted all my life.

But I've realised in the last short time, no matter how bad that action might have been, or how big the regret I hold about doing it, if I am genuinely sorry for my action, there is nothing stopping me from letting go of that regret. Other, that is, than my need to keep berating myself, my need to keep that particular guilt or shame alive, which is all pretty pointless, a waste of energy and time... in fact, boring!!

I'm going to pause for a drink.

Ah, that's better.

So, after years of berating myself for certain actions, I have chosen to let it all go. Phew! Pity it took me to die before I really realised the waste of time taken up with regrets... but never mind... I got here! And as for anything else... every single experience, no matter how big or little... wonderful or ghastly... has made me who I am at this time of speaking. And I really like who I am... in fact, I love who I am now. I have even come to grips with genuinely loving... and not just giving lip service... to my wrinkles and droopy breasts. Good Grief, Gaia... what are you doing? Funerals and breasts do not go together.

But, the way I see it, children dear, is that if I can write about God and Sex in the same sentence as I did in Genitals, Sex and Other Bits and Pieces, then I can talk about my breasts at my funeral.

Anyway, in talking about breasts, my lovely friend Pat is going to talk next about what she had in mind when she made the wonderful green work next to my coffin. When I first saw my naked, moulded, 66-year-old breasts, I must say, I thought … 'Oh dear... not a good look.' But as I allowed myself to see the whole picture, I began to see the magnificence of the whole being.

The glory of that which is I.

The exact glory and magnificence of that which is you.

So, as for my friend, cancer... yes, cancer has truly been my friend. I have been glad to walk hand in hand with this energy that so many people fear. It has shown me aspects of myself that I had no idea existed in me, and which had no reason to appear without something as extreme as cancer coming into my life. I compare it to the trees in Australia that need the brutality and horror of a bushfire to allow it to reseed itself so it can re-appear again in all its magnificence. The burning of the dross. The letting go of what is, to allow the joy of what can be to enter.

And yes, the physical pain of cancer has been brutal at times. And the thought that cancer could bring all sorts of gross experiences to me before my physical life ends is not nice to think about. So, I don't.

Please don't feel sad that cancer has been the reason for my leaving. I left at exactly the right time... not one minute too early or too late. No matter what the physical reality of my death, know that my soul was filled with joy and belly laughter.

My spirit was full of peace. My being was full of love for you all."

These words from Gaia and this piece of art demonstrate profound intimacy with the human form in all its expression. Gaia's art came with me when I came back to Australia after 20 years in New Zealand. My art is an expression of my encounters with humanity. It is multi-faceted, as we all are, yet society has honoured only sport and academia, never bringing full honour to all our expressions. My encouragement in sharing this story is to foster you sharing your story and vulnerability during this time. This intimacy with Gaia has been balm and salve for me through my own troubled times, and my world view has been changed by association.

When we share this full expression, this is what we receive.

A colleague wrote, "The joy you bring to others will have greatest impact to those who are open to and want to receive it. What you showed me last night was profound. How privileged I am to have seen your work. It was profound intimacy with the physical being of human form. Your gift to others is to be hands on with them in art; to make them art; to give them art; to show beauty when doubt exists."

Joyful empowerment is ours when we can fully appreciate the gift of our humanity.

Pat Armitstead is no stranger to grief and loss. She lost her home and business twice, is a cancer survivor, endured a violent relationship, avoided bankruptcy by repaying $80,000 in 2 years, had 10 car accidents in 18 months (none her fault, so she says) and plummeted when her partner of 20 years left with another woman. She says, "My life's work has been a series of devotional appointments with my higher self, and like Stephen Jenkinson I have come to see that grief is a skill of deep living, which enables us to recognise the world's suffering. It is also the midwife for being able to fall in love with being alive again."

Pat's grieving workshops are about restoring a sense of wellbeing and supporting people to be fully self-expressed through finding meaning in life events. She has been described as a Spiritual Midwife, delivering people out of the darkness.

Multi award-winning speaker, facilitator, author
Past president of the National Speakers Association NZ
Speaker of the Year 2002, NSA NZ

Mental Health in the Workplace
Conscious and Transformational Leadership
Humour, Engagement and Wellbeing

0487105785
pat@joyology.co.nz
Skype: Joyologist
www.joyology.co.nz

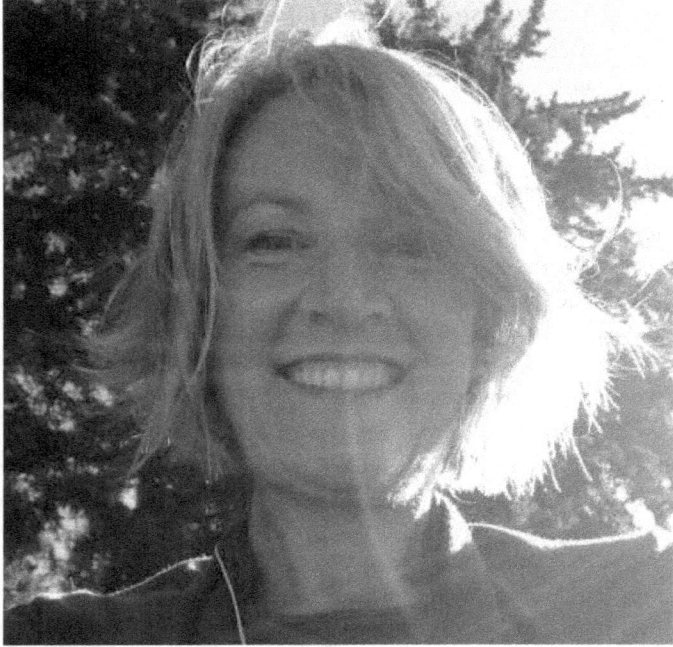

Seventh Story

By Melissa Turnock

I am 50 years old. I once had breast cancer and now I am ready to support women like me who have finished treatment and are finding themselves back in their old life with no sense of self, not sure who they are or what brings them joy. I have found my purpose through the discomfort and gifts of breast cancer, and I am ready to serve women just like me, so they don't need to feel as lost as I did.

In December 2009, when I was just 41 years old, I intuitively did my first ever breast self-exam and found a lump, a grade three breast cancer (BC) that pressed a dramatic pause on my life as a Pilates Studio owner and mum to an 8-year-old. The next 9 months of life was all about being a cancer patient; the next 9 years have been about healing from what lead to me getting BC. That has now evidently become my soul's purpose and is the work I bring to the world. Well, to the women of Sydney, anyway. But you know, anything seems possible with the internet.

December 2009, my week looked like this: first time ever (truly really) breast self-exam and I found a lump in my left breast on Monday, biopsy for Wednesday, and by Friday I was sitting in front of the surgeon saying, "Hi, so do I have cancer?" The next week was the start of surgery, a lumpectomy. And then the news that there was more cancer lurking in there, and so now a mastectomy, all lymph nodes out and chemotherapy were on the cards. That all ended in October 2010 with a get out of jail free card because they were very happy they had got it all.

As a woman with BC you are part of well-oiled machine, just as it should be given the huge numbers of women that get it: 1 in 8 in my part of Sydney, last time I read the stats. Therefore, thankfully, there wasn't one moment in there that I wasn't exactly sure what to do next, who I needed to see, where the rooms were or how to navigate the system. It was very well supported, thank goodness. You even get a BC nurse to support you, too. The only decision I had to really make was do they take one breast or two, and which day did I want to lose my breasts, Thursday or Friday? With very little fuss over lunch in a coffee shop at Hornsby Westfield, I chose a double mastectomy and reconstruction, all in one procedure. The ever-practical Aquarian, happy to do as much as I could in one go as I sure as shit didn't want to come back here again if I could help it. I have not for one minute regretted the enormity of that surgical procedure. It only took me 4 weeks to get full movement back in my arm – that I credit to my Pilates knowledge. I was able to prepare my body for the procedure(s) and rehab myself, too.

Getting reconstruction is a slow process as you have to gradually enlargen the implants, but those frequent visits to my surgeon were a very supportive part of the process as I felt someone cared, got what I was going through and was overseeing my recovery. She was a she, and that meant a lot to me; how could a man possibly understand the significance of losing breasts, right? I am now the proud owner of recon boobs. I got some amazingly real nipple tattoos in place last year and I'm pretty darn happy with how they look, in and out of clothes.

So, why did I get cancer? I think – no, I know – the journey of breast cancer began as a child, learning to block down my personal expression, living in a family where resentment and unhappiness was silently brewing under the surface of a quietly composed miserable couple. I have memories of desperately trying to make them happy, fielding complaints from one about the other, dreading Christmas because we all had to put on the happy face and I could see how forced it was. There was no space for the emerging me or how I felt as I grew, no one ever really asked me how I was, so my tender-aged response to that was to shut down and stay well behaved, not express much that might rock the boat and make them even more unhappy. Funny thing is, when you are a kid, you don't know any different, you don't have a whole lot to compare to so you just get on with it. Our home was generally an icy atmosphere, no one saying what they really thought, tolerating each other. That was not a place of safety or ease for me to be me. And having two younger brothers meant I was protecting them as much as I could, too.

Once the treatment is over you assume you will feel elated, wonderful, and so full of life, as you have beaten cancer. But it was then that the wheels fell off. I found myself hiding in my car crying, avoiding going home as I felt so sad, full on grief as the loss. There is such expectation that after cancer you will be over the moon, and for me there was a lot of guilt in that not being the case. Everyone is so pumped for you that you've done it and keep saying, "You must feel amazing." In truth, I sank into a deep hole that saw me visit the GP; he of course offered me antidepressants. That was a big NO.

Months of chemo fill you with such a disconnect to your body, such a feeling of not wanting to feel, not wanting to be in this body anymore, that I instinctively knew that getting back into my body was what was now needed, not more numbing out. I asked about counselling and learnt about a mental health program that offered a few sessions with a Psychologist. And she was great, just what I needed to help me reframe my perception of my new body. I couldn't even look at my breasts in the mirror, I was filled with such distaste for these white mounds masquerading as breasts. I found ways to avoid undressing in front of my husband as I was so embarrassed. As you can imagine our intimacy went out the window and still to this day is such a challenge for me. I was dumped into full on menopause as a result of the chemo, and that is NO fun either.

Looking back, I believe my years of pre-cancer meditation helped me enormously during my treatment, gave me the opportunity to almost watch my treatment from an arms distance. I knew it was just my physical body that was being ravaged by surgery and chemo, not the real ME. Not the one that would eventually pull me out of that mess and bring me to this point.

Quite intuitively, and perhaps being guided by something much greater than me, I was led on this inner journey, and still continue to walk that path. Firstly, I spent three weeks alone in a small village in northern India, committing to three hours of mediation, movement and self-enquiry every day before I left the room for what became brunch. That was when the tears started to flow. What followed is 8 years of looking deeply within me, trying every tool, reading every book, practicing everything I could to uncover the beauty of the woman that lurked underneath the surface presentation of Melissa Turnock, the person that the world got to see.

What I have unearthed was a child that never got to express herself, was never seen as an individual with a voice. I have spent hours with this child, many versions of my inner child, hearing her, soothing her, showing her that she did matter and that she was the strongest, bravest kid that got me though all of that, BUT the important part was that I didn't need to live my life from that place of lack or fear anymore. I have been able to reframe the way I acted, the beliefs I had about myself, the censorship of the real me.

It's so interesting to me that my first career was as a Speech Pathologist, working with people that have lost their ability to communicate clearly. Two career paths later, I am now working in the area of emotional embodiment, bringing our emotional selves to the light and offering a way for us to safely see, feel and release them from our systems. When we bury our emotions, our stuff gets locked down and the body holds that tension. It gets held and held until the body can no longer hold it, and something stops us in our tracks. For me, it was breast cancer, a wake-up call that my body was unable to keep going as it was.

I now work with women in my BodyWisdom sessions and use TRE (or trauma release exercises), guided meditation, intuition and energy work to let go of parts of ourselves that are keeping us in a place of fear, sadness or lack of self-worth. It is such an honour to support women in this way now and show them the many ways to trust their bodies again, to see for themselves that emotions are messengers that can be safely felt and released. And the magic that comes after they are released, such as wisdom, self-love and recollection of who you truly are, finds its way to the surface. Life begins again, our new normal. A richer, more whole version of us.

Melissa's dream is to offer workshops, retreats and online webinars to women who have had breast cancer, to bring us all together, to teach simple tools to help with managing your emotions and start to empower women to take healing back into their own hands.

www.bodywisdom.com.au is her website and she encourages any woman that wants to reconnect to themselves post-cancer or anyone who knows a woman like that to share her work.

She lives in Newport, Sydney, looking out at the water every day, and she loves so much about herself: her body's capacity to heal, and her heart's capacity to grow through what has been offered to her through her cancer experience.

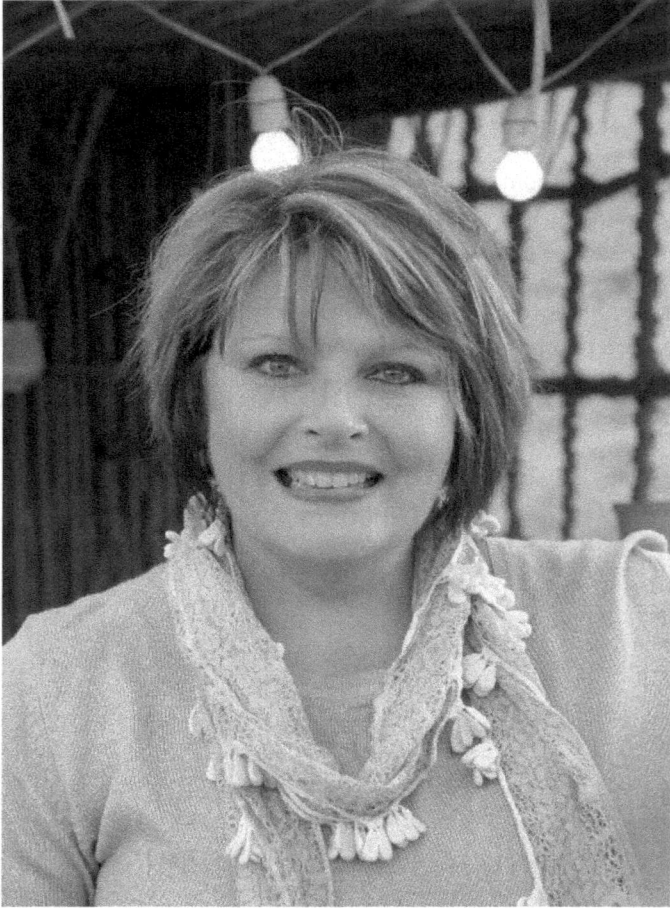

Eighth Story

By Sue Woods

It's going to be okay, darling.

On Monday 22nd of December 2008, I laid in bed after waking, running through the never-ending list of things that had to be done before Christmas that was only days away. I wasn't feeling like the manically festive elf that I was every year. Instead, I just felt tired, I felt weary, I felt like my heart wasn't really in anything and I wasn't sure why. The thought of all I still had to do was overwhelming, but nobody else was going to do it, so I told myself to get up and get over myself and get at it.

The years leading up to this point had been an awful time for our family. My mother in-law was diagnosed with bone cancer, and in her 18 months of suffering before she passed my every moment was spent caring for her. I was working full-time, running a household, my daughter Anthea was still in high school and it was stressful. Two weeks before she passed in 2006 she handed the baton on to my own beautiful dad who was diagnosed with lung cancer. I found I was revisiting the same chemo and radium wards, going to the oncology and specialist appointments, asking the same questions over and over and all while trying to hold myself together at work, at home, for the kids, and for my parents, who were facing the biggest battle of their lives.

My dad lost his battle on the 6th of March 2008 and my mother dropped her bundle of life. She didn't cope, she just broke, so I supported her. It was an exhaustingly painful time after we lost dad. As I lay in bed that Monday morning reflecting, I acknowledged to myself that this was in all likelihood the reason for my melancholy. It was our first Christmas without dad, and I believed that this was why my heart felt heavy and I was fatigued.

As these thoughts skittered gently in and out of my mind I suddenly had a thought that seemed to scream with its intensity. I couldn't remember when I had last checked my breast for lumps! I was always so diligent every month as my nana had lost both of her breasts to cancer. I tried to think when I had last checked and I couldn't remember. My life had been so out of control caring about everyone else that I had totally forgotten about performing such a basic and vital task. What the hell was wrong with me?

So, I pulled my pyjama top up and raised my right arm above my head and started gently feeling around. And there it was. Under my nipple and a little to the left was a long, sausage shaped mass. How in the name of God could I have not felt this before? It was huge! As I probed further, I realised that this insidious sausage shape also had 2 tiny pea-like lumps sitting beside it. I lay in bed staring at the ceiling with tears running down my face and into my ears. How could this possibly be happening to me? How was I going to tell my husband and the kids? My daughter was going to be in year 12 next year, I didn't want to be sick, I didn't want to die, I was a good person, oh my God, how is mum going to cope with this? I dragged myself up and sat on the side of the bed and broke my heart. I shuffled through the house like a broken old woman and rang my doctor. My lady doctor was on holidays and I had to book in with someone I didn't know. I felt shaky, like I was in shock, the ball of dread sitting in my stomach was aching. The phone rang and it was mum. She rang to say she had had an awful dream the night before. She dreamt I had breast cancer. I placed the phone gently into the cradle when the call had ended and made my way unsteadily into the bathroom to get ready for the doctor.

That night, I told my husband, son and daughter that I had found a lump in my bust but not to be worried as I just needed to get it checked and it would probably be nothing. I told mum and kept it as upbeat as I could – I didn't let her know about the size of it. I told no one how afraid I was. I couldn't upset them with my fear.

The GP agreed it was a very sizable lump. She called the breast clinic. I was in between mammograms, which everyone agreed was a good sign. Because of the time of the year, I had to wait until the 9th of January to have a mammogram. Then I had to wait until the 16th of January for an ultrasound. As soon as the ultrasound started it was like a panic button had been pressed and the room filled with nurses and specialists. A core biopsy was needed from a few places in my breast. I knew something was so wrong, a nurse held my hand and I said to her, "This is bad, isn't it?" She replied that yes it was, but they didn't know how bad yet. She tried to engage me in conversation to take my mind off what was happening and asked what I was doing for the rest of the day. I told her through my tears that it was my birthday – I will never forget the look of sadness and pity that radiated from her face. I spent the rest of my birthday laying on my bed with 3 ice filled condoms in my bra crying inconsolably.

On the 20th January at 10am, my husband Ian, Anthea and I were ushered into an office at the Breast Screen Clinic at Chermside. I always remember the room was a strange triangular shape and Anthea had to sit at the end of the desk. The doctor entered with a nurse and they both sat down. As soon as I saw the nurse I knew it was bad news – they wouldn't be sending her in to give me a high five and a "well done, get outta here". There were no informalities or pleasantries to start, it was right to the point.

The doctor said that, just as she had suspected the week before, I did indeed have a huge malignant tumour in my right breast. She stated that because of the size of the tumour compared to the size of my breast that I would require a complete mastectomy. The tumour was invasive as it had gone from within my milk ducts into my breast tissue. The tumour was aggressive, I would require chemotherapy after the surgery, I would require radiation therapy after the chemo. I would definitely lose my hair. I had an appointment with a professor up at the RBWH. She handed me a wad of paperwork and a couple of DVDs to watch about having a mastectomy and reconstruction. As she spoke, the weirdest thing happened. It was like she was being sucked backwards into a long hallway and was getting smaller and smaller. I could see her mouth moving and I could hear what she was saying but I just couldn't comprehend that it was me she was talking about. I turned to Ian and saw the tears streaming down his face, I looked at Anthea and she was sobbing and being hugged by the nurse. I remember trying to stretch over to Anthea to comfort her and I couldn't reach but I kept saying it's going to be okay darling, it's going to be okay. The doctor then asked if I had any questions about anything and I just shook my head.

I picked up all of my information sheets, appointments and movies and left her office. We walked through the automatic doors out into the blinding Summer sunshine as if in a trance – we were silent. Ian went around to the driver's door and I went to hug Anthea to comfort her and found myself breaking my heart on her shoulders. I cried unlike I had cried before, heaving guttural tears, I knew I shouldn't be doing this to my daughter but I was crazed. Slowly I became aware of a sound like an animal howling, a primal noise of pain and fear. Ian had come around the car and grabbed us both and I realised then that the howling had come from me. My son Matthew called on our way home to see how I had gone. I didn't want to tell him over the phone so I asked him to come home. He knew straight away that the news was bad. My beautiful 20-year-old burly son arrived home and cried on my shoulder. As a family we made a pact that we would get through whatever lay ahead of us together, and when it was over we would be stronger than ever.

Then, the rest of the world had to be told. Mum was in Tamworth and flew home. She arrived on my doorstep and fell into my arms and I was the one patting her on the back and saying, "It is going to be okay mum, we will get through this."

The house was swamped with visitors, family, friends, the kid's friends and parents. The scans were pulled out over and over, everyone wanted to see what breast cancer looked like. The day after I found out one of my sisters brought over an inflatable bikini top that she had found on the front of a Ralph magazine. She jokingly said that I could make myself as big as I liked! I didn't think it was funny and put it into the bin after she left. Flowers arrived daily, the phone didn't stop ringing, loved ones baked and made meals, mum moved in, I was placed on numerous prayer lists, we got Anthea a puppy to help her cope. I was supposed to be going back to work, and had to tell them I would have to take a year off.

I felt like I was on some crazy fairground ride that was going faster and faster and I couldn't get off. And while all this was going on I was keeping the smile on my face and saying, "I am going to be fine, this is not going to beat me, I am a fighter." Never, ever would I show what was going on inside my head, not to anyone. The fear was a physical being, it was a pain that didn't go away, it radiated from my gut and filled every part of my body. I would wake in the night sobbing, my pillow drenched with tears, and I would find myself standing at the doors of Matt and Annie's bedrooms as they slept, literally wrapping my arms around myself to hold the pain in. I prayed as I looked at them, dear God let me see them get married, let me see them grow into the adults they would be, let me see my grandbabies be born, let me get through what I had ahead of me.

I got my acrylic nails taken off – that could cause infection. I went and got my teeth checked – that could cause infection. I had a bone scan and a heart scan so that the specialists had a base point to work with as the aggressive chemo they planned could damage my bones and heart. I needed to have a sentinel node biopsy. This is where a radioactive dye is injected into the tumour and the first lymph node that it drains to is your sentinel node. At the time of surgery, they remove the sentinel node and test it to see if there is any malignancy, and logically if there is none there then it would mean that the cancer hasn't spread to any other lymph glands. As I lay on the metal trolley awaiting this test there was a kerfuffle as the staff couldn't find something. I asked the female doctor what they were looking for and she replied they needed an ultrasound machine so they could find the lump. I took her hand and placed it on the large mass within my breast and she just looked at me and said, "Oh, my darling."

On the 20th of February, 2 months after I discovered the lump, I finally went in for my surgery. My name was called and I had to leave everyone in the waiting room. After showering and dressing in a mauve hospital gown, pressure socks, and paper booties and hat, I was placed on a bed to wait. As I waited, I prayed, I spoke to dad, spoke to my nan, asked them to watch over me and keep me safe, and I cried big sobbing tears that ran onto my paper hat. Suddenly, a face appeared at the end of my bed – it was a teacher from the school that I worked at. She coincidentally had an appointment that day as she was going through her own cancer battle and had enquired as to where I was and had just made her way in. Angela held my hand and walked with me up until the doors of the operating theatre. I will never ever forget that feeling of gratitude that I had for the human contact of someone I knew at that moment of my life.

I awoke in the ward to see a sea of worried faces surrounding the end of the bed. I could share with them the wonderful news that the cancer had not gone to my lymph nodes. Later that night a nurse got me up to go to the toilet and I haemorrhaged and passed out. I woke up on the floor with the drip trolley beside me and asked if I had fallen out of bed.

The following morning, I had to go and have a shower, and the nurse asked me if I wanted her to come as I would be seeing my wound for the first time. I replied that I would be okay as I had seen what my nan's chest looked like after her mastectomies. I took my nightie off and looked at myself in the mirror. I started shaking and could not stop. The wound was just covered with a strip of tape, but it wasn't the wound – it was the empty space where my breast used to be. My chest was concave, I stared in horror at the nothingness. I recalled all of my comments prior to this moment of how my breasts had done their job and fed my babies and how I was worried about losing my hair more and thought to myself I knew nothing about how I would feel at this moment.

I came home with the drain still in. The hospital had supplied me with a lovely pink floral bag to carry the drain around in. I had to monitor how much blood I was still losing and tag and change the drain container every day. After a few days at home I became feverish and in an incredible amount of pain. My mother insisted I go to the doctors and I ended up being taken by ambulance back to hospital with a life-threatening infection. I recovered from that only to pick up a gastro bug a week later and be admitted once again. I finally got the drain removed when I was in hospital the second time and was finally able to throw that bloody floral bag away. My beautiful breast care nurse, Patsy, made me a little cotton insert filled with wadding for me to tuck into my bra, to "give me a little bit of shape," she said. I couldn't believe such a simple thing would make me feel so much better about myself.

Once my wound had healed and I was feeling stronger it was time for my chemo to start. I went and got a wig whilst I still had hair for when the inevitable happened. At my first round I sat in the recliner chair and watched as the nurses covered themselves in protective clothing and began pumping the poison into my body. By the time it was finished I was swollen up like a balloon, and my pee had changed to a pretty peach colour. I went home with a cocktail of drugs for the coming days. I went to bed and then awoke in the early hours feeling violently ill with a headache unlike any I had had before.

After two weeks, I noticed my head was feeling sore, and if I touched my hair it hurt. On Sunday the 19th of April, I woke before anyone else in the house and went in to have a shower. As I stood under the water I noticed on the floor of the recess a tuft of hair. I gazed at it in horror and slowly raised my arm and ran my fingers through my hair. I looked in disbelief at the hair that sat in my palm. I started pulling at my hair and found to my despair that I could pull the hair from my scalp with the same energy and sensation as tearing fairy floss apart. I kept tearing and tearing the hair from my head and watched as it piled up in the corner of the shower. Finally, I could pull no more hair out and I was spent. I stepped shakily out of the shower and gazed at the monstrous sight before me.

I had strange tufts of hair still attached randomly all over my head. I reflected that I looked like the characters of a movie I had once seen about a group of people that had survived a nuclear holocaust. I stared at my head, I stared at my chest and I found myself cowering at my vulnerability and nakedness I now had to face the world with. I slowly dressed and wrapped a towel around my head and went to wake Ian. I roused him in tears and he gently asked me to show him, I couldn't look him in the eye as he looked at my mess of a head. He put the towel back on and told me that he still thought I was beautiful. Then, he told me to go outside and he went in and cleaned my hair out of the shower recess for me. My sister came over with her clippers and shaved the tufts off and I wore a bandanna for the first time. Mum said that now my hair had fallen out she was going to go back home.

My life now had a strange routine – week one of chemo I spent laying on the lounge feeling incredibly ill. Week two, my immune system would bottom out and I could go nowhere and have no visitors. Week three, I would start to feel like my old self and would be in a frenzy of getting the house in order and preparing meals for when I would hit rock bottom again.

Ellen became my best friend; I would make myself get up in the afternoon and put a bit of makeup on because I didn't want to scare the kids with how awful I looked. My eyebrows and eyelashes fell out. I tried to experiment wearing my wig. It wouldn't do a single thing I tried to do with it and my hairdresser told me to drop it off to her. I went into her salon and she said she had taken it home, washed it and let it run around her back yard until it got its crazies out. She cut it while it was on my head and I then could go out and look relatively normal and not in a scarf where I was obviously a sick person. I started having night sweats and hot flushes and found out that I was now in a chemically induced fully blown menopause.

I finished my 6 rounds of chemotherapy and then had to start my 25 rounds of radiation therapy. In a horrendous coincidence I found myself allocated to the same radium room and bed that my dad had used not even 12 months before. Every time I laid on the bed I would gaze at the same ceiling he would have and imagine him there. I spoke to him every time I had a treatment. My friend Angela, who had met me before my operation, was having radiation at the same time as me, and we used to make sure we would put the gowns we had to wear next to each other just as a comforting reminder to one another. I thought, first of all, that the radium was a complete walk in the park compared to having chemo – strip off, pop the gown on, lay on the bed as the machine circled around you, and it was done. But, as the treatment went on, my skin on the wall of my chest went from looking and feeling a little sunburned to the flesh across the scar like rotten meat with a consistency of jelly – I would have easily been able to poke my finger into the wall of my chest. I had to dress it with an expensive cream that people in the burns unit used and cover it with a bandage.

Then, one day, just like that, my treatment was done. After spending nearly a whole year up at the hospital and it and the staff feeling like home and my second family, I was on my own. My oncologist told me I would be taking Tamoxifen for 5 years and visiting her every 3 months. I got teary talking to her one day about feeling afraid now that I was on my own and wasn't being constantly checked and tested. So, she thought it would be an idea for me to go and speak to a psychologist. I'll never forget walking with Ian and seeing the sign for the psychology ward and saying to him, "I can't believe I have ended up here." A tiny woman greeted us and asked me to explain to her what lead me to her room. I explained that I felt like I had been through a meteorite storm, that I had been hit and hit and hit and gone from one awful battle to another, and then suddenly I had gotten through the storm and had hit nothingness – I was floating and floundering on my own with nothing to hold onto. After I had poured all of this out she looked up from her notebook and said in her soft, calm voice, "and how did that make you feel?" I answered, "shattered," to which she nodded sagely and wrote it down. At that moment, I looked at her and thought she could use that for a title of a book: *Shattered – One Woman's Recount of her Battle with Breast Cancer*. She then advised me to go for more walks. As we left the building

Ian told me, "Not to worry Suey, there's nothing wrong with you."

I had my breast reconstruction 18 months after I finished my treatment. I had a trans-flap procedure where they use the fat from your belly and create a breast from that. I did this solely and wholly for me, so that I could feel womanlier again. Whilst I am so happy with the results, I could never do it again. It was a 14-hour operation, and because I had had so much anaesthetic, I vomited and vomited. What was worse was because I couldn't brace myself I was literally just vomiting all over myself. But, I healed and recovered and felt so much more confidant in myself. I was offered the option of having a nipple made and then tattooed with colour to make it look real. I declined this because my tummy that was now my breast had the stretch marks on it from being pregnant with my babies, and I wear them with pride.

I diligently continued to go to all my check-ups with my oncologist and my radiologist every 3 months. Then I was allowed to go every 6 months. Then, on one of my routine check-ups, my oncologist told me that I was considered a very high-risk patient for my cancer to return. She told me that I had to stay on my medication for 10 years rather than the 5 that I was initially told. As she flicked through the pages of my file I saw for the first time on the cover page of every section was a sticker with large red letters saying **HIGH RISK PATIENT**. As I sat there, I felt like my body was made out of a house of cards and it was just crumpling in on itself. I left my appointment feeling broken. How could I have never seen the stickers before? I thought I only had a couple more years of taking the Tamoxifen, now I had 7 more years. Nobody had ever said I was a high-risk patient of my cancer coming back. Jesus, when is this ever going to end?

I came home feeling stunned and feeling not right. I went to work and my colleagues were asking me if I was alright and I told them I didn't know. When I was home I just stayed in bed. I felt sick at heart, it was a physical thing, my whole being was filled with dread. I had a total breakdown of relationship with my mother which rippled to my sisters as well. I couldn't explain what was wrong with me as I didn't know – I had tried to explain this to my mother that I didn't know what was wrong, but that I knew it had something to do with my cancer. I reached out for help with my old GP who had become a counsellor. Together we worked to get me back to being me. The mind is an extraordinary thing and for me, even though I believed I had coped with everything that had happened on my cancer journey and had done it with a positive attitude and a brave smile on my face, when I saw the HIGH-RISK sticker, that was the trigger that caused my mind to shut down.

I have recently celebrated being 8 years cancer free. I am 15 kilos heavier than I started out, thanks to the side effects of taking Tamoxifen. I never forget to check my breast and have my mammogram every year. I have been able to support many friends and strangers with advice and information after they have been diagnosed, and am very happy to show anyone that is thinking about reconstruction my own right breast complete with beautiful baby stretch marks. Right from the year of my treatment, my dear friend Carmelina (whose sister is a breast cancer survivor) and I have run fundraising events to help find a cure.

Right from the moment I was diagnosed, I was carried away on a wave of love and support from everyone in my life. At first, I was overwhelmed, as I am the one that normally is the carer or giver, and I found it uncomfortable. Then, I consciously decided that I was going to soak up every visit, hug, phone call, meal or gift and let all of that love give me the strength to get through what I was going through. The people in my life that supported me through that year will never know how much it meant to me. My family and friends rallied around and surrounded me with a force field of love that I will never forget the feel of. I am so grateful and so blessed to have them in my life.

After going through this I am still the same, but very different. I now know that worry is a wasted emotion, as is sweating the small stuff. If I am stuck in a traffic jam, I now admire the colour of the sky and think that this is exactly where God wants me to be. I relish and treasure the beauty that lies in everything and am very mindful about taking moments and views deep within me. I listen to my body and rest when I need to. I use all my good stuff all of the time because I am worth it. I burn the special candles and use the fancy soaps that have been given to me. I nurture myself by having regular massages and getting my nails done. I practise kindness always and stay away from negative situations and people.

Throughout everything, my husband Ian and my children Matthew and Anthea have been the constants in my life that made me fight so ferociously. They have, and continue to, surround me with their love and protection. We have faced losing one another and come out the other side with a strength and bond that can't be broken. I have been able to see them grow into strong, caring and beautiful adults. My daughter is going to be moving into a new house she has built next month, and my son and his lovely partner are going to be giving me my first grandbaby in August. Ian and I are rock solid and are so overjoyed about the next exciting chapter in our lives together.

My life is good.

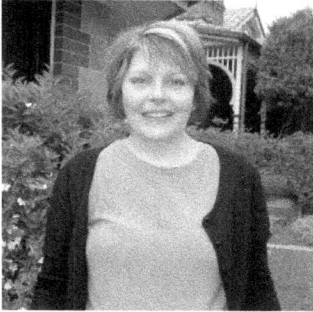

Sue was born and bred in Brisbane. She attended Hendra High School and then studied at Seven Hills College of Art. She worked in the jewellery industry for many years and then changed careers and has been employed at Education Queensland for the last twenty years. She has worked in Learning Support, Behaviour Management, Special Needs and Administration and has volunteered as a Pyjama Angel with children in care to help develop a love of learning.

Sue has a love of reading, travelling, painting, the theatre and arts, exploring antique stores, movies, dining out and meeting with her Book Club every month.

Sue lives on the north side of Brisbane with her childhood sweetheart husband Ian whom she met when she was 16 years old. She shares her home with Eddie the Toy Poodle/Bichon Frise, who she says saved the family when she got sick.

Sue has two adult children, Matthew and Anthea, who are, in her opinion, her greatest achievements and sources of joy in her life.

Sue and Ian have just recently become "empty nesters" with Anthea moving into her recently built first home. Matthew and his beautiful partner Adriana are due to have their first baby in August. Sue is quite beside herself at the thought of becoming a first time Nana and having another family member to love.

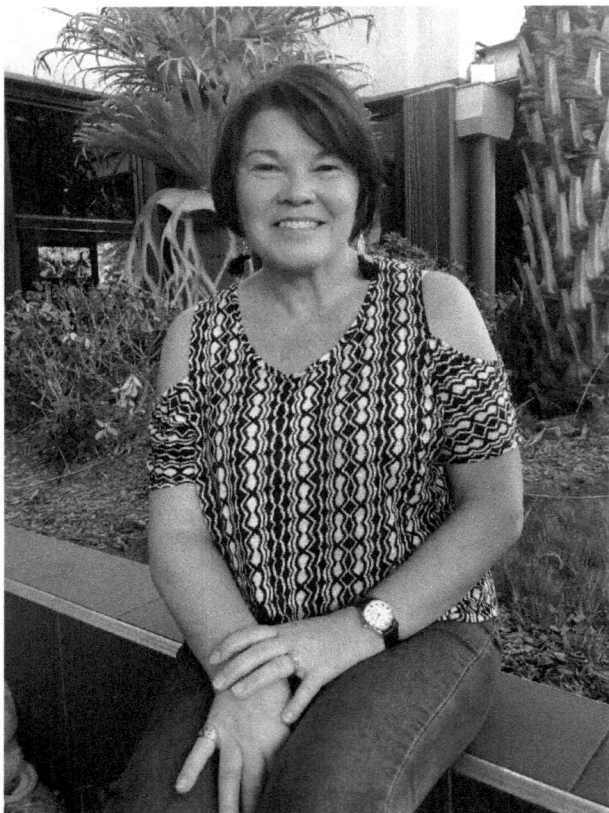

Ninth Story

By Jeanette Murray

I was a travelling sales manager. I was away a lot travelling all over Queensland and part of New South Wales, and I'd be gone for a week at a time. That was all I was: always busy. In addition, I had my own sales agent business which was me selling to retailers, so I worked on commission for 47 different companies in Queensland.

So, there I was, 51 years old, when my husband pushed me to go to my doctor, who said to me, "I want to do a full medical. You've gotten to that age where you're maybe premenopausal, and we just want to find out where you are in life."

However, I was constantly busy, and it was about 6 or 8 weeks later that my doctor said to me, "Well, you are going to go and get a mammogram and an ultrasound." He was sending me to the women's imaging and diagnostic centre because he believed that we just needed to get a full body scan and do a check-up.

I'd just come back from a trade fair and I thought, 'Ok, you're pushing.' Then my husband was saying, "That's it – you're not going to work tomorrow. You are going to go and get this done."

So, I finally went, and I thought everything was fine. Then, the doctor came out and said, "Look – we're not sure about what's happening here. We want you to stay." I said, "I can't stay, I've got appointments to go to; I'm sorry." She said, "You've got no choice – you're going to have to be back here in the morning!" My response was, "I'll see what I can do." That was my attitude because I didn't feel anything. I didn't know anything was wrong, so I thought, 'OK, I'll come back in the morning.' Even that night I didn't think anything of it – I was too focused on my business and my busy life.

I went back and had to have a biopsy. I'd never had one before and I didn't know what I was in for. So, I was lying on the table and the nurse was there with me, and the doctor was so good. She did the biopsies and then I sat in the coffee shop at St. Andrew's Hospital feeling really overwhelmed with the whole thing. I had a coffee and just sat there for a few hours because I couldn't drive anywhere, as I was not feeling fantastic after the anaesthetic from the biopsies. I finally went back to work – I had to go to the Gold Coast, and the next day, a Thursday afternoon, my doctor phoned me. I remember I was leaving Coastal Kitchen and Cutlery, and I was in the car and he said, "There's no other way to tell you this, because I know you're not going to come back, you will be too busy to turn up!" He said, "You have breast cancer. I've already rung the surgeon, and you are booked in to see him Monday. You've got no choice, you will turn up." My attitude until then had been, "I'll be fine, I'll be right, no problem with me."

I had to drive back from the Gold Coast to Brisbane, and I rang my husband who immediately fell to bits. I had to go and tell my daughter, and I rang my son. Telling my daughter was the hardest thing I've ever done; I didn't know to what extent my breast cancer was and how bad it was. The doctor had said to me that they're pretty sure they got it early, but they don't know to what extent. So, I had to keep everyone together because they were all falling apart around me and I was always the strong one; I had to put on the brave face and keep working and being like, "I'm fine, it's easy, no problem; you know we're going to be fine, I'm not going anywhere."

I saw the surgeon at 9am on the Monday, and they said they couldn't get me in for a couple of weeks because they were booked out. He said, "No, we can do better than that – you'll be here Friday morning at 6am." Well, in between the Monday night and Thursday night I went out west to Toowoomba Chinchilla Dalby and visited all my retail stores, and they couldn't get over the fact that I just been diagnosed with breast cancer and I was still working. It was my business, I had to keep working, and it kept me busy and kept the family focused on other things, not on me at home thinking about "What's Friday going to bring?"

Friday morning: I ended up at the counter checking in to the Mater Hospital, and I broke down; my husband wasn't coping really well either. I pulled myself together and I had to leave Ken in the waiting room. I went in, and the young nurse had the right sense of temperament and humour to keep me focusing on things the right way instead of having a total mental breakdown. I said, "I don't want to wake up until you got it all – I don't want to be woken up and find out I've got to come back in again and have more taken out because you haven't got it all." So, they kept me under and I had two sections taken out. They sent off the sections in the blood tests, and I didn't wake up until they got every bit. They also removed 6 of my lymph nodes, and I was so lucky that it hadn't travelled at all. I was only in hospital overnight, however when

I got home my dressing was coming part and I nearly fainted in the shower. I had to go to the chemist to get some more bandage and rebandage it.

It all felt like being on a roller coaster ride: you just don't know how you going to get off, when you are going to get off. You don't know what's going to happen tomorrow, you don't know and you're scared because you don't know if you are going to get breast cancer back.

I can't remember March; in April or May I started radiation therapy. I didn't have to have chemo because it hadn't travelled to my lymph nodes. People don't realise chemo doesn't stop anything – it decreases the size of things. It decreases your chances of getting breast cancer back, but it doesn't stop what is happening now.

I was really, really lucky to catch it so early. It wasn't my normal mammogram procedure – it was only because I going through life and hormonal changes that my doctor insisted I do a full medical.

So, I'm having the radiation therapy, and again, you don't even know what you're in for. You get little tattoos so when you go in and have radiation they have the exact spot where you have radiation therapy. You can't wear your normal deodorant, you can't wear this, you can't wear that. Nobody tells you any of these things; nobody told you what you're in for. 38 days of radiation. I would get dressed and go to work every day, and then have the radiation every day, and I got so tired. One day,

I was so tired that I went to walk out with the hospital gown on!

I'm on the table having radiation, and you feel like you are just a body to them. It's normal for them; it's something they do every day. It's not for you, because you're the one that's had breast cancer, you're the one lying there going like, 'What the hell just happened to me? Why is this happening to me? What did I do to the universe or to God for this to be happening to me?' You're on this ride that you're just trying to cope with every day, and you have to go to work.

I was told, "So many business women going through breast cancer are doing what you're doing every day and they're wondering what happened to them and just trying to cope every day. They've gone from being on boards and running companies to 'How do they keep going?'." "You are not who you used to be." "You have this stress level to cope with and challenge you, your mind is gone into overload and you still trying to function on a daily basis the way you always have but that's changed." "You don't get back to where you were before."

I was trying to keep going the way I always had, kept pushing myself to cope with being on radiation treatment and not being well because of it. My whole life been turned upside down. Most of my companies were supportive, however one turned around and said to me, "Your figures are down." After all that I had been through, I sat there totally stunned. I was so angry that within a few weeks I sent him a letter telling him in a very nice polite way to shove it.

One day, I got in the car and I started to cry, and I said, "I can't do this anymore." I threw away a lot of a big income because of that, and that's when life was turned upside down for me. It wasn't just about breast cancer, but also my job and my career. Everything I had done since I was 32 – and that's about 20 years of everything – I threw out the window. I couldn't manage it mentally or physically.

I'm now 58. I've gone through a lot of changes. In those six years, I've got my real estate certificate. I found I don't like being just a real estate person, and I am very artistic and like to renovate.

Everyone said to me "you know how to dress", so I opened up a fashion boutique I had that for 3 years. I opened it up not knowing that the shopping centre was not a good shopping centre anymore, and my business didn't survive. In those years, I went from a very high income, to absolutely no income, to losing my business, and losing everything. When you go through breast cancer, you change the way you think; you find that things are not as important as people. People are so much more important. I couldn't care less if I lived in a tin shed out in the sticks. We lost everything we lost our home – the banks tied the shop and the home together. I didn't have the knowledge, and I didn't have the experience.

Now, I have a lot more experience, and I try to pass it on to people just starting out through the chamber of commerce.

I fundraise every year for breast cancer. It started 3 years ago when I had the Boutique. At that time, I was part of a two-year research program on your body and how it changes after breast cancer. So, I gave myself 6 weeks to organise a Pretty in Pink high-tea fundraiser which is supported by Pine Rivers Bowls Club. I raised two-and-a-half thousand dollars that year. Last year, I had it again – it was in May. Last year, in May, it was a sell-out that raised $6,980 that went to Breast Cancer Network Australia.

This year, it's in October. I have partnered with Be Uplifted, which is 100% run by volunteers. The board is an independent board, and the founding director is a breast cancer survivor. Be Uplifted is an organisation that gives support to families and to those going through this, including men. They give daily support: if you've got kids that need to get to school, or if the dad that may have fallen to bits and just can't cope, they are there. They have volunteers that go out and actually help with the daily stuff. They provide the service for free, because we all need to help each other.

As a woman, a mum, a sister, a grandmother – whatever age you are, your health is the most important thing. Don't go along the rest of your life and think that 'I'll be right, nothing happens to me.' Know your body and everything about it and go for your medical check-ups. Even at a young age, know your body, because breast cancer is happening more and more in the young.

It has been 6 years since my breast cancer was diagnosed and I've had the five-year all clear and am off medication. I can't do and be the way I was again. I wanted to be part of my daughter's life and my grandkids' lives, and now I can pick the kids up from school. I can be there for them.

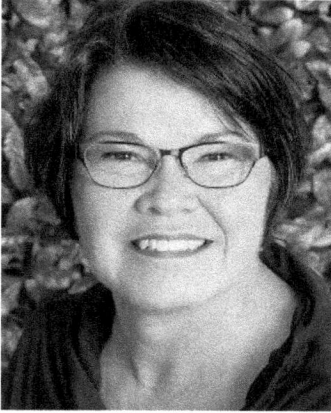

Jeanette Murray is a property stylist, interior designer, sales woman, customer service specialist and more. She is also a fundraiser for various breast cancer charities.

She is a survivor in more ways than you would think, but not just a survivor – she believes, no matter what, in being positive and forever giving back to others, as that makes her feel awesome and worthwhile.

A mother to 3 wonderful adults that she wouldn't trade for anything, step-mum to 3 more, a grand-mum to 8 who she treasures enormously, a wife to Ken. She has married 3 times, and she thinks that the extreme levels of abuse in her before-life may have caused the cancer (who knows).

Jeanette is a professional sales person who has worked in retail either in a store or as sales management travelling all over the country. But now, she has given herself permission to follow her love and dreams to go back to study and complete an interior design degree so that her passion of creating will come to life. She may never have done this if it wasn't for getting breast cancer, but who knows, one thing she does know is that life does change in many ways from the day of diagnosis, whether you want it to or not.

Ph: (04) 5818 1000
Email: hello@keylime.com.au or Jen.45@bigpond.net.au

Jeanette is North Brisbane based but will travel.

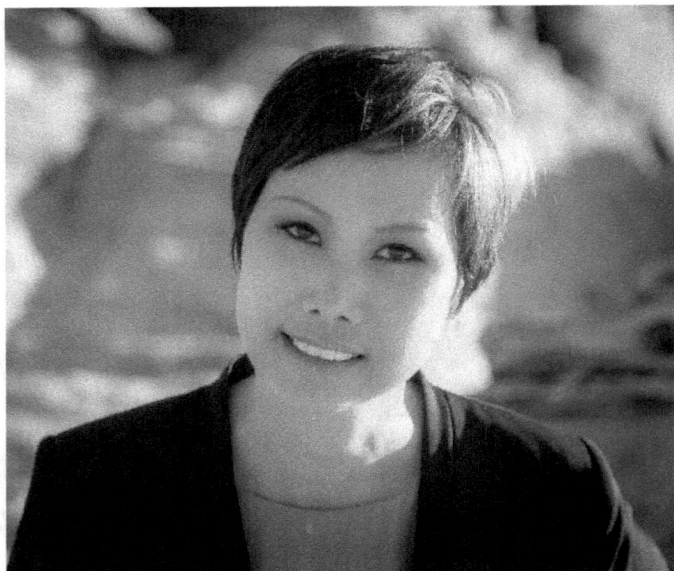

Tenth Story

By Heidi Yi

Life was good. I enjoyed what I did, running my cosmetics company and looking after my regular customers. I maintained a busy lifestyle and frequently travelled interstate for my business, as well as working for others.

I ate out a lot on the go, drank lots of coffee to stay focused and had no time to exercise. I didn't like public transport so I chose to drive everywhere, resigning myself to the stress of being stuck in Sydney traffic, trying to get to places on time.

The hard work was paying off. I was winning business awards.

And then I got a cold, which was unusual for me. I was 34-and-a-half years old and hadn't had cold in years, so why now?

I put it down to the weather, it was winter, after all. But that cold stayed around for a month, it really knocked me around.

Then came a new symptom: chest pain.

I went to my GP, and as was the protocol for anyone with suspicious chest pain, they sent me to the hospital emergency department for further assessment. The usual tests were run: bloods, an ECG, a chest X-ray, and when they all came back normal I was discharged home.

A new month dawned and with it brought entirely new sensations in my body – the source of which were investigated singularly and dismissed due to their seemingly unrelated nature.

A nose bleed... they happen.

Back pain – it was excruciating… and as I'd had a recent hard fall on concrete, it made sense.

General 'tiredness' – hey, I was running my own business, volunteering at charities whenever time allowed, and had a strong social network to keep up with… who wouldn't feel tired?

Only in hindsight did these, what appeared on the surface to be, unrelated sensations reveal themselves to be symptoms of something larger. However, at the time I started to feel a growing awareness that I was complaining more and more often that I wasn't feeling well.

This awareness brought me to the consultation rooms of various doctors in my quest for answers; the most extreme of which was a spine MRI to make sure I hadn't broken any bones when I had fallen. With each doctor's visit, the tests were coming back normal, which – although reassuring – resulted in no change to how I was feeling.

Something kept telling me things weren't right. I started to think it was all in my head, but deep down, knowing my body, I believed there truly was something wrong.

So back to the doctors I went, just in case. I started getting second and third opinions from different doctors. As I was going from one doctor to another – telling each one of them the same story – I couldn't help but feel like I was being a hypochondriac trying to get a 'diagnosis' which didn't exist.

My biggest fear up to this point was that I was going to have a heart attack. So, with that fear abated, I decided to move on. Besides, by this time I'd used up a lot of medical resources, and, being reassured there was nothing wrong with me, I let it go and got back to work. I didn't want to be known as 'that patient'.

Furthermore, a common diagnosis started to emerge from the multiple doctors.

I must be run down. Bed rest was needed.

Some doctors even went so far as to put it down to anxiety. For that, I was reassured all was okay, and to take it easy. If the pain persists, come back.

Late one night, whilst lying on the lounge watching some TV after a long week, I felt a sharp, painful lump on my left breast. It was the size of a golf ball.

One week later, on 2 December 2013 – only a month after I celebrated my 35th birthday – I was diagnosed with breast cancer.

I sat in the doctor's office as he delivered the news. I didn't panic. I didn't know what to do, so I asked him if he got my name right on the report. Could we redo the test, just to make sure it wasn't a false positive reading? I'd had an ultrasound and a biopsy which, he informed me, confirmed breast cancer.

Really? It couldn't be true?

Okay, so it wasn't a heart attack. But at my age, cancer didn't even cross my mind. I thought cancer was something people get later in life – like 50s or 60s. I hadn't heard of people many having breast cancer in their 30s.

My body froze in disbelief as the first lucid thought that came to mind was, Am I going to die?

I started to feel the distress well up inside me, but there were no screams, yelling or crying. As the doctor explained the treatment involved, I sat silently numb. As he reassured me that things would be okay, I was hearing him delivering a death sentence.

How long have I got? And how was I going to break the news to my parents when I can't even digest the news myself?

Was this the cause of my symptoms and me being unwell for the past six months? Or did I get the cancer because my body and immune system were comprised because I had been unwell?

I could have had cancer for as long as six months and didn't even know it.

The next few days passed in a blur. I started the carousel of phone calls... marking the start of my two-year breast cancer treatment.

I temporarily retired my business and informed all my customers that I was going on a medical break.

I made an appointment with a breast surgeon. Being so close to Christmas I was very lucky to find one located near me and be seen within 72-hours of diagnosis.

My biggest lessons in life were taught to me during my double mastectomy, radiotherapy, chemotherapy, targeted therapy with Herceptin, hormone therapy, and later breast reconstruction.

I also had multiple complications, both physically and emotionally. I had a reaction when beginning chemo, breaking out in a rash. And when I started to vomit severely during the chemotherapy, I knew that things weren't going to be easy. I had chemo-induced menopause, bringing on hot flushes, infertility and with that, my dreams of one day having children.

My dignity plummeted as I grieved the loss of my two breasts.

I was told I would lose my hair. But when was that going to happen? I would check every day thinking, is it going to be today? Then the day finally came. After having couple of rounds of chemo, it hit me. That was the day when I saw rest of my hair falling out in the shower.

From the barrage my body had been under, I couldn't drive for a while and felt I'd lost my independence. I am not the type to ask people for help.

And due to the chemo, I had two life-threatening infections. One was Neutropenic Sepsis, where your white cell count becomes very low. With a compromised immune system this is considered a medical emergency. During this time, I became very anaemic and required a blood transfusion. I was admitted to hospital in isolation for a week in the cancer ward and required intravenous antibiotics.

To make things worse, I started getting abdominal pain and severe diarrhoea. Because of the strong antibiotics used during treatment of the Neutropenic Sepsis, I had developed C difficile colitis. The good bacteria in the gut were killed off by the antibiotics, leaving a toxin-producing pathogen called Clostridium Difficile to cause havoc. I had to be treated with yet another course of antibiotics and a week in hospital.

All up, I had over 20 hospital admissions and close to 10 operations. I remember one occasion, whilst being prepped for surgery, an anaesthetist saw my familiar face and said, "You are back again!"

I said, "Yes I am back, your repeat customer!"

I have a strong family history of cancer but thankfully the BRCA1 and BRCA2 (BReast CAncer) gene mutation came back negative.

Through this experience, I have felt what extreme pain was like. When someone divulges to me they've been through breast cancer, my honest response is, "Yes, I have felt your pain."

Once I started getting better and regaining my health, I felt so thankful I was starting to live my life again. But this time I was going to turn things around.

Prior to cancer I liked working hard to earn a living so I could start saving up for my future when I retired. I was making lots of sacrifices by working hard, staying up till late to reap the rewards later. Maybe it wasn't a good idea as I had actually brought retirement forward by having cancer.

The whole experience has made me appreciate the things that I had taken for granted. I feel I've been given a second chance at life, so have made some dramatic changes including my diet, lifestyle and enforcing a work-life balance.

These big lifestyle changes are to prolong my life and live that life happy and healthy. Now, looking after myself means putting my health first, work second, and everything else can wait. Because if I don't put my health at number one, everything else will fall apart.

I don't stress or sweat over small stuff anymore. Lesson learnt. And I have set boundaries by learning to say no to things that will make me stressed or exhausted. If I am not available, I am not available – full stop! I used to get upset or easily offended if someone said or did something; now I have learnt to brush them off and move on as I have more important things to take care of.

By staying committed to this, I have become a better person. I now have less commitments, I love my sleep-ins, I say no to things that take up too much of my time, and I spend more time with friends. I take my time getting things done, in my own time, when I am ready. I am no longer time-pressured.

I have joined a gym and have a personal trainer to help me keep fit. I am more aware of what I eat by reading the food labels and avoiding processed foods. I try to cook more and eat more fresh fruit, vegetables and drink more water.

I feel like I am a winner and I don't need to win awards to get recognition for that. I fought cancer and to me, that is a big achievement on its own.

I am enjoying life and treating today like it is my last day. I have written myself a bucket list – all the things I want to do in life, and to my surprise – I have ticked off 80% of them! One of the major ones that got a big tick was writing more books. I had started writing books in my spare time while recovering because I found it quite therapeutic.

One of them was a memoir, called The DeTerminator – From Powderpuff to Chemo, my personal account of my cancer journey. You can find about more about me and all my books at www.heidiyi.com.

Lastly, my biggest wish from my experience is to help empower others, regardless of gender, age, whether you have a family history or not, if you think something is not right, listen to your innermost self and put that as your priority.

Heidi Yi is a self-published author and cancer survivor, and this is her story. She was diagnosed with: Invasive Ductal Carcinoma Grade 3, HER2 positive.

You can reach Heidi at www.heidiyi.com.

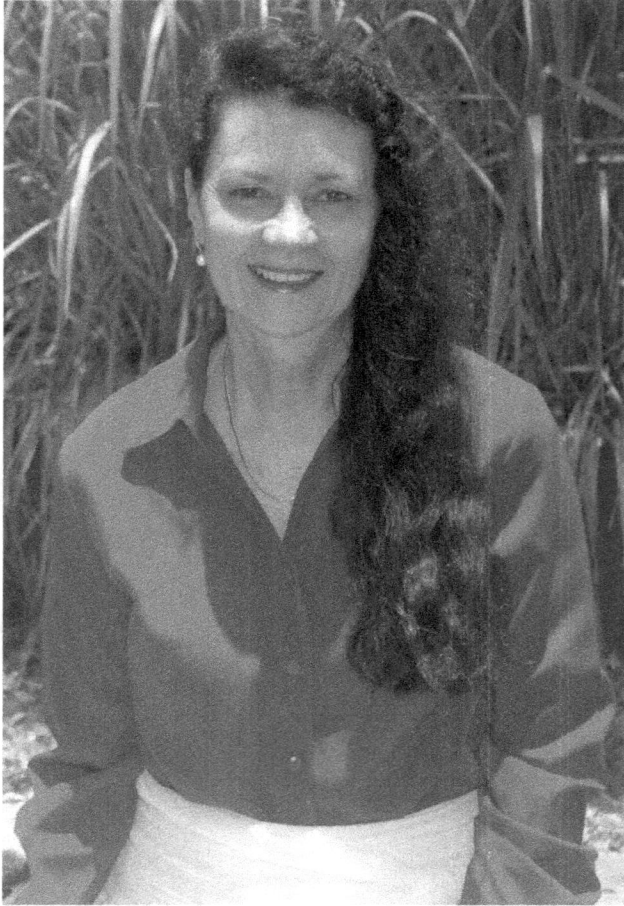

Eleventh Story

By Karen Alexander

Surviving breast cancer is easy!

The purpose of putting my thoughts and events to paper is to inspire, educate and bring hope. To help another person struggling with a fear of what to do and how to be rid of the disease in her body called cancer, and to give an awareness of many options available.

I speak from many years of experience and am a walking, talking encyclopaedia when it comes to cancer. I survive the epigenetic way. A different approach to what I first thought or knew when I was originally diagnosed with breast cancer in 2003.

When I first started out, I thought by doing what the medical system and doctors told me was the way to beat cancer. Therefore, that was the direction I took and where I relied on for my hope. Unfortunately, I was to learn a much larger lesson, and a very ugly lesson it has proven to be.

I was a career woman, loved my working life, also a wife and mother. Holding an MBA specialising in Project Management, a qualified Justice of the Peace and did support work for domestic violence victims. I held high moral and ethical values and this was my downfall. I was an overachiever and a perfectionist.

By January 2006, the cancer had spread into my bones and I was riddled with cancer. My vertebrae broke in two places, and I was faced with a life crisis of learning how to walk again on top of the insurmountable thought of how to beat the cancer. The PET scan showed cancer activity in the following sites: C6, T1, T2, T3, T5, T6 and several right and left ribs, sternum etc, etc. The side effects of the drugs had me accumulating over half a kilo in fluids a day. I was told repeatedly by medical doctors and staff to get my affairs in order, and with the letter written by the oncologist we purchased my burial plot.

I was broken physically, mentally, emotionally and almost spiritually.

I followed my intuition, and that was not to have chemotherapy. I would not have that poison in my body. I did try some other drugs, but the side effects weren't letting my body heal. They were causing a domino effect where I was being prescribed more drugs, which caused more complications and none of the results from tests were telling me there was any improvement.

The trust in doctors and medical science came to a screeching halt when I researched some drugs they had me on. One was called Tamoxifen[1], listed on the US Government Toxicology website as a human carcinogen and known to cause liver and uterine cancer.

This was a betrayal for me in epic proportions. Remember, I had not only blindly believed the doctors were there for my

---

[1] https://ntp.niehs.nih.gov/ntp/roc/content/profiles/tamoxifen.pdf

wellbeing, but it was also where I had misplaced my hope of getting better. I only had myself to blame.

I battled getting off a synthetic drug called Dexamethasone going through depression and tears by the bucket full. It was the hardest drug to ditch, as being a steroid, it masked the pain. It took me 18 months to rid that drug from my life.

When the porta Cath became blocked and had to be removed in 2008, that was the last time I ever subjected myself to a hospital.

Reflecting upon the despair and fear at this point in my life, I penned the following in my journal many years later when I focused on healing, the emotional trauma and to try to find closure.

DESPAIR

I had to learn the true raw meaning of hopelessness and
despair
To find the very essence of courage
Through the reflection upon the Fear...
True Fear grips the soul and squeezes...
So you become a pawn in someone else's plan.

You become like a ball of clay in the potter's hand,
To mould you with their beliefs,
That does not belong to your soul.
The colour of this Fear is blackness.

Even a moonless night still leaves the traveller
Stars to guide them on their quest.

There are no Suns, or Moons or Stars,
there is only emptiness
and like a blind person
trying to feel their way down an unfamiliar corridor

You learn to trust yourself,
Your intuition is the only guidance you can rely on.
With the belief and a conviction that, eventually
The fear and despair will fade
And you will be left with courage
To continue on your quest in life.

I made the decision to walk away from the medical system. I learnt to follow my intuition on what was right for my body. Little did I know at the time this is a common gift given to people in similar predicaments and commonly penned and known as the "intuitive healer". It had come to my rescue when I had no one turn to. Many work colleagues and friends said their goodbyes. They only knew that once you were diagnosed with terminal incurable cancer, then there is no hope.

No Hope was all I was given for years, to the extent that to block out the negativity and beliefs of others. I became a recluse for nearly nine years. Rarely did I leave my home, and when I did it was with my husband because I needed help to do the grocery shopping due to the damage and weakness in my vertebrae when lifting the shopping bags.

I am proud to say I can again do the grocery shopping alone!

I learnt about resilience, endurance and willpower, and I learnt how to fight.

Fighting for the right to live.

At the 5-to-7-year marker since we purchased my burial plot, I struggled through survival guilt. I felt guilty when heard the news about people dying of cancer or someone heroically raising funds for cancer research in their last-ditch effort. This led me to learn another valuable lesson.

Everyone who has ever been diagnosed with cancer has sat in a doctor or oncologists office and received the news. It is at that very point everyone has the freedom of how they choose to fight the disease. It comes down to your philosophy in life and your belief systems. If you believe that medical science is the answer, then that is the path you will follow. If you choose the epigenetic life like I have and that is your belief, then you are free to make that choice as well. I stopped being controlled by other people's fears a long time ago.

I have very dear friends who watched silently while I took matters into my own hands. They didn't know what to do. An excerpt from the poem they wrote and sent to me last year titled Karen (2017) can give you an insight into the emotional heartstrings of friendship.

"We doubted you then, but you started to fight
And shamed us with ardent desire
To beat this cruel fiend who was taking your life
And to do so with commitment and fire.

No easy task when doubt was in place
In the minds of your family and friends.
They could not help; did not know how,
But you proved them all wrong in the end.

We could but watch and offer support
Respecting the decisions you made,
And give you space to heal yourself
When everything else had failed."

Everyone has their own path to follow when it comes to fighting any type of cancer. No one has the right to tell anyone what to do if they have not had experience in this area.

It is now over 12 years since we purchased my burial plot, and it has been more than 10 years since I walked away from the medical system, where I had blindly put my hope and trust. During this time, I have found that I never did need that mastectomy. In the past 10 years there is not one product or item I have been able to claim on Medicare or the Private Health Fund with regards to cancer. All I needed was the right knowledge, a belief in myself, and to find healing in a nurturing environment.

Remember — cancer is only to be understood, not feared.

In the early days, it was the positive thinking and willpower 80% of the time to overcome the fear and doubts I faced every day, on whether I would survive, and 20% focused on foods and what to eat. After about five years, I had overcome many of my doubts and fears and focused more on fine tuning the foods and food combinations. So, there was a switch on 20% mind and 80% focused on foods. I made rules and stuck by them; below are three:

Rule 1 – Nothing out of a can or a packet (processed foods)
Rule 2 – No Soy
Rule 3 – No Sugar, dairy or alcohol etc. etc.

In 2017 I became an entrepreneur and wrote my book. The purpose of the book was to inspire others and to let them know what options are available if they choose to fight the epigenetic way. It also proved to give me closure on a very emotional traumatic experience.

My blog is receiving hits from around the world, and it is a great comfort to me. To know someone in the world is receiving confirmation and knowledge they are not walking their path alone when it comes to fighting a disease surrounded by so much fear and greed. I have noticed people's eyes light up when they hear my story. I can give hope where no hope is usually given. I live my life with courage and conviction.

Born in Queensland, Australia, Karen spent eight years of her early childhood in Papua New Guinea. When her family returned to Australia, she finished her school years in Toowoomba, in Queensland.

As a young adult, she spent three years as a governess in the Queensland outback near Julia Creek, Charters Towers and Longreach.

When she married and settled down, she spent 13 years living in mining towns in Central Queensland. She had her own consulting business for three years before the diagnosis of incurable terminal cancer in 2006. This journey of surviving cancer has taught her:

- *how to heal,*
- *how to find peace, and*
- *how to become the person she was always meant to be.*

She holds an MBA (Master of Business Administration) specialising in Project Management and a Professional Certificate of Wellbeing Coaching & Management.

Author of Terminal Cancer – How I Survive
Contributor to Your Well-Being – Phoenix Edition
Contributor to Telling Your True Story

Website:
http://courageandconviction.life
Facebook:
https://www.facebook.com/courageandconviction/

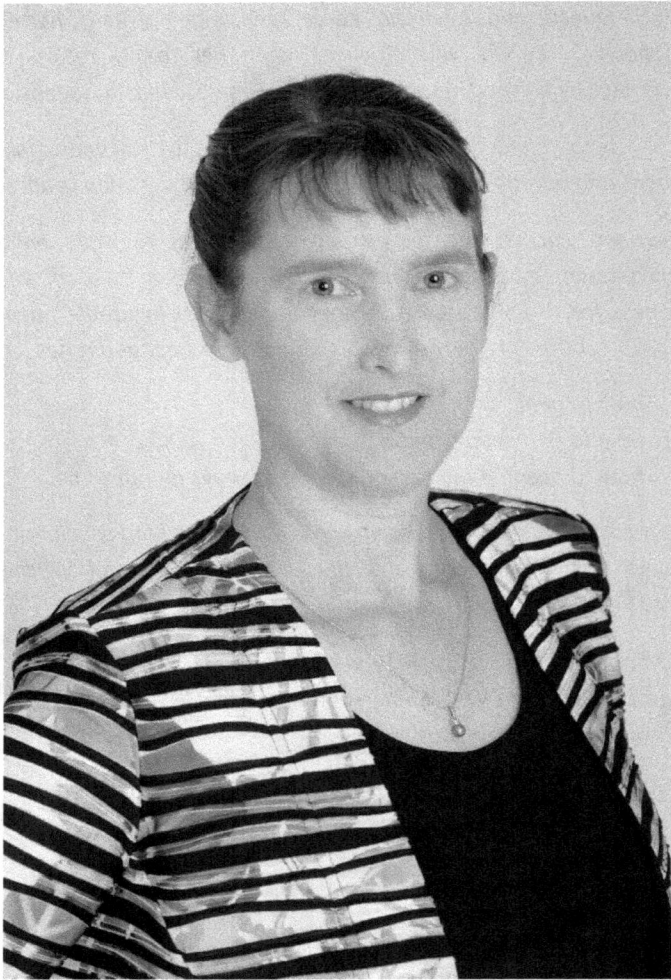

Twelfth Story

By Jay Anderson

I have been "touched by breast cancer" in two ways... firstly, I am a professional involved in supporting people who experience a range of life challenges – my background is in counselling and psychology. I see adults and children with a range of concerns or difficulties. I provide counselling for the Cancer Council in a country region.

My clients are people who have cancer, or partners, family or children. I provide one-on-one private counselling sessions. A large number of my clients are women who have been diagnosed with breast cancer. The ages of the women vary, as do their experiences. I am also involved in presenting to groups (cancer clients and families) regarding wellbeing, psychological impact and emotional health.

I provide therapeutic support and counselling. Many women are also going through various levels of treatment. So, sessions can involve discussing emotions and experiences. Many women are overwhelmed and distressed. They appreciate the listening ear of an independent person who can assist them to process their emotions and be there with them along their journey.

Women with breast cancer have a range of concerns. For some, it is the grief and distress associated with the diagnosis. For others, it is the stress and anxiety of treatment. For many women, it is the fear of dying – a common situation for many people in our community. Other women worry about their children, partners, family... and then for other women it is the recovery and life afterwards... the wondering about whether the cancer will return and the ongoing tests to see how their health is going. Some women have a changed outlook on life, influenced by their cancer diagnosis – this may not be understood or valued by their partner, friends or family. An altering of attitudes, beliefs and plans for life can occur – and this is often a point of contention amongst those involved.

As we know, for anyone, the diagnosis of cancer is a shock. It brings with it so many emotions that can be hard to process or to understand. Many people around the person have difficulty understanding or knowing how they can help. This means that they may not help, or not be involved, or they may be very supportive or they may just say things that are not helpful at all. This can be most challenging for the person at the centre of it all – the woman who has breast cancer.

A woman's body is often the source of mixed emotion – a topic that affects her self-esteem and self-value. Throughout her life, her body may be something that she either appreciates or dislikes. Her breasts are a key feature and discovering cancer in this part of her body is a more public experience that presents its own challenges. Many other common cancers are internal to the body – and there is not such a visual impact when treatment involves surgery. Often the treatment for breast cancer will involve significant impacts to a woman's breast. The visual impact for a woman is one that will affect her daily as she views her body and her identity. Some women are comfortable with the concept of losing a breast in the understanding that it may save their life, while for other women this is a most distressing situation. There are so many psychological and emotional effects of breast cancer. It is a complex scenario that is so individual and experiences differ greatly.

The incidence of breast cancer in our community seems more prevalent. It certainly has gained wider public understanding and people are more likely to share their diagnosis or experience with others. This can assist those involved in a number of ways. Public figures involved in fundraising or in their own cancer experience can assist those with their own cancer journey to get through this challenging situation.

In my role with women, I use my listening skills and therapeutic skills to assist them to work through their particular situation. We undertake a range of things such as reflecting on their life, re-evaluating values, beliefs and relationships, sharing and processing emotions, managing grief and reactions or daily life experiences involving anxiety or depression. I am privileged to participate in the life journey of women in this situation – I share their journey with them, engage and connect with them in their experience. I value every human being's life and experience, and women who have breast cancer I am able to interact and connect with on many levels about many issues. I am in awe of the commitment and focus that women have to those around them – worrying about their loved ones often before themselves. We are able to process this and their emotions and discuss strategies to manage all of this, as well as considerations for self-care so that they can look after themselves and their own wellbeing during this part of their life journey.

I assist women to find themselves, to find purpose and meaning in their situation. Women are able to process emotions, reflect on their life and their future, and experience peace… there are a range of therapeutic techniques that are beneficial – and it can vary from person to person as to what techniques and strategies will suit each individual and each situation.

To women out there who are not engaged in counselling or therapy, I encourage you to access a service as it can provide great benefits. You can contact your local Cancer Council, or the APS (Australian Psychological Society) has a "Find a Psychologist" service.

I encourage all women to spend some time getting to know their true self. Being comfortable with who you are and your body is important for your wellbeing. Being aware of and reflecting on the components of wellbeing is also important and beneficial. Check out the PERMA model by Dr Seligman, the five pillars of psychological wellbeing and happiness: Positive emotion, Engagement, Relationships, Meaning and Accomplishment.

Many people don't realise that all these things are so important – this practical information comes from the **Positive Psychology field** involving the study of human flourishing. Some Professionals call it:

The Pleasurable Life – (Positive Emotions)

The Engaged Life – (Flow & Mindfulness)

The Meaningful Life – (Meaning & Purpose)

In summary, the PERMA model is an excellent model to be aware of to assist in understanding self, your current situation and your future, in how things may be different.

Positive emotions – feeling good

Engagement – being completely absorbed in activities

Relationships – being authentically connected to others

Meaning – purposeful existence

Achievement – a sense of accomplishment and success

The SAHMRI Wellbeing and Resilience Centre proposed PERMA PLUS, where they added: Physical Activity, Nutrition, Sleep and Optimism to measure and build wellbeing. So, these are all aspects of your wellbeing to reflect on and consider.

The second way that I was touched by breast cancer is on a personal level – my brother's mother-in-law was recently diagnosed with breast cancer and has since passed away. Our two families have been connected for over 20 years, and so the impact on many individuals has been felt. A range of emotions and experiences involved… many people reflecting on a life well lived, a woman's connection across so many people – positive memories and experiences.

Our culture can find death and dying a challenge. It is often a topic not easily considered or discussed. As human beings, we are often "doing" much more than we are "being". Having the opportunity to reflect on life and one's future is important, and I encourage everyone to spend some time in reflection and contemplation, and the PERMA model is an excellent framework for this process.

Jay is a registered psychologist, counsellor and play therapist. She practices in southwest Western Australia at the South West Wellbeing Centre. Jay has worked in the human services field for about 20 years, of which the last 10 have involved therapeutic work. Jay's passion is "making a difference" and she works with adults as well as children. She has a strong interest in animal assisted therapy and her dog has engaged in therapy with her for a few years now.

You will find Jay at www.swwellbeing.com.au.

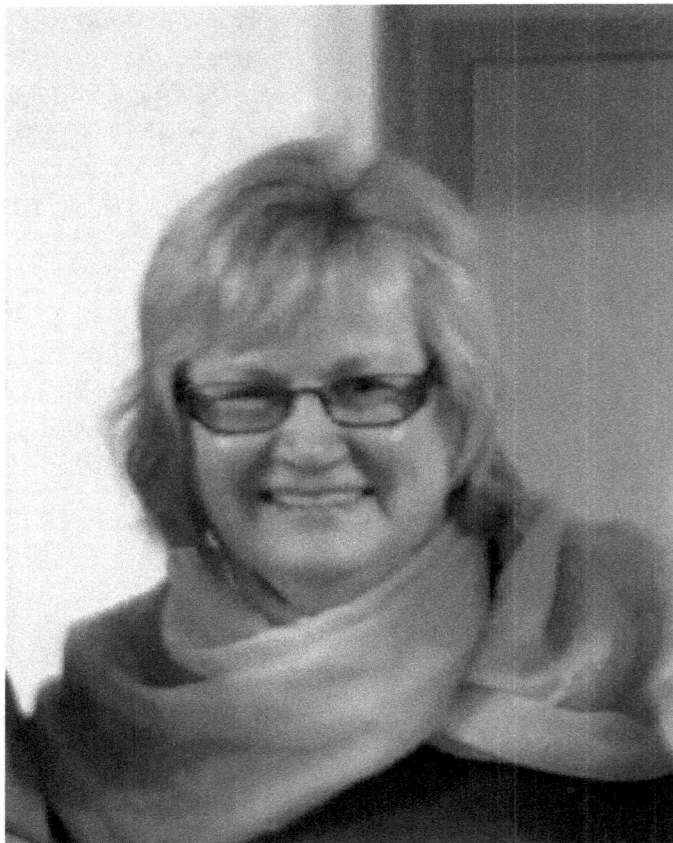

Thirteenth Story

By Rita-Marie Lenton

To begin my story on how Breast Cancer has touched my life, I would have to go back to June/July 1992 when we had just purchased our first home and were moving to Margate to live. The family was excited and looking forward to a new start. Everything came to a crashing holt, however, when in the early hours of the morning 1st July 1992, our phone rang.

I still can see my husband David sitting in total shock as he listened to his mother on the other end of the telephone, telling him of the most horrific, catastrophic news regarding a triple fatality that had occurred within the family. I felt so helpless as I watched my husband have a minor breakdown in the days and weeks that followed. It was hard to bear.

At the time, my mother-in-law, Betty, who had recently been diagnosed with bi-polar, fell into a deep depression. Over the next couple of weeks, she came to visit us in Margate from Cairns, where we could assess her condition for ourselves. This is when we realised how much she needed help. The family all agreed that mum should move nearer to us, so we sent mum home to Cairns so she could prepare for the move.

We managed to find mum a new place in a retirement village near to us, but as it was a new village we had to wait for her villa to be built. We had a great time planning her new home but when the day arrived that she could move into her villa she had another episode of depression and came back home to stay with us.

For the next six months we played "visit the villa" in the hope of getting mum ready to stay in the villa full time on her own. To say this was exhausting would be an understatement, but "what the hell"? It's what families do.

Twelve months had almost passed since the tragedy of death in the family. Betty was still living with us most days of the week. I still remember the morning she came out of the bathroom and asked me to take a look at her breast as it felt sore. From the moment I laid eyes on her breast I knew we were dealing with breast cancer. I contacted our doctor that morning who told me to bring her straight in. She examined mum and sent her straight away for a mammogram. The doctor also requested we return straight away with the results, and when we got back to see her, she had already made an appointment for Mum to go and see specialist immediately. The specialist didn't muck around, either. He took a biopsy and asked we come back for the results on the following Saturday morning, the 3rd of July.

As mum sat clutching my hand, the specialist delivered the news as gently as he could, but my mind went blank as he told mum that she had full blown breast cancer and needed to be operated on as soon as possible.

At this point, mum piped up and said, "Can the operation wait until Monday?"

The specialist responded "of course!"

"Good," replied mum. "It's Rita-Marie's birthday today, and she deserves to enjoy the rest of her day." Bless her.

Breaking the news to rest of the family was another chore that fell to me. Everyone was upset, of course, and asked what it was about the 3rd of July that we had to hear bad news every year. As I sat there agreeing with them, I was screaming inside my head, "For God's sake, it's my bloody birthday." I got a bit caught up in "why me?" in the moment.

Mum's surgery was scheduled for Monday morning, and David and I sat at the hospital waiting for the surgeon to come and see us. He broke the news that the cancer was worse than first thought. Mum had a total mastectomy of her left breast. All the lymph nodes were removed and the cancer had also impeded the chest wall, resulting in most of the muscle being taken away.

Once her surgery wound healed, mum started 6 weeks of radiation therapy & physiotherapy to get her left arm moving again. This meant daily visits to the Wesley Hospital, and I am certain my car went there every day on autopilot.

On her weekly visits to the physiotherapist I learned how to do lymphatic massage on mum daily so that her arm didn't swell; at the same time, I was taking care of the family, so I was really starting to get tired myself.

Through all this, mum's depression started to lift, and we found she could stay in her villa a few nights a week. There was a light at the end of the tunnel.

With the help of her community support group Grow, mum was able to face her breast cancer front on. It was as though it gave her the will to live again. She slowly improved, not only overcoming her depression, but she had survived the breast cancer and she went on to enjoy living in her retirement village, telling us constantly that it was the best time of her life. She was an inspiration to us all.

How was I touched by breast cancer? I was lucky to have had a mother-in-law that was grateful I was there to help her, and I feel blessed that we had time to grow close together through some pretty heavy and trying times.

Mum's favourite part of the Grow program was "Constant Improvement", and she lived it every day to the end.

Do I believe that the tragic death contributed to my mother in law's breast cancer?

While I don't believe the tragic death in family was the sole cause of Betty's breast cancer, it certainly was the reason we didn't pick up on it sooner as we were busy dealing with her deep depression over the deaths within the family circle.

You can connect with Rita-Marie Lenton on her Facebook page:
https://www.facebook.com/soulcrystalearth/

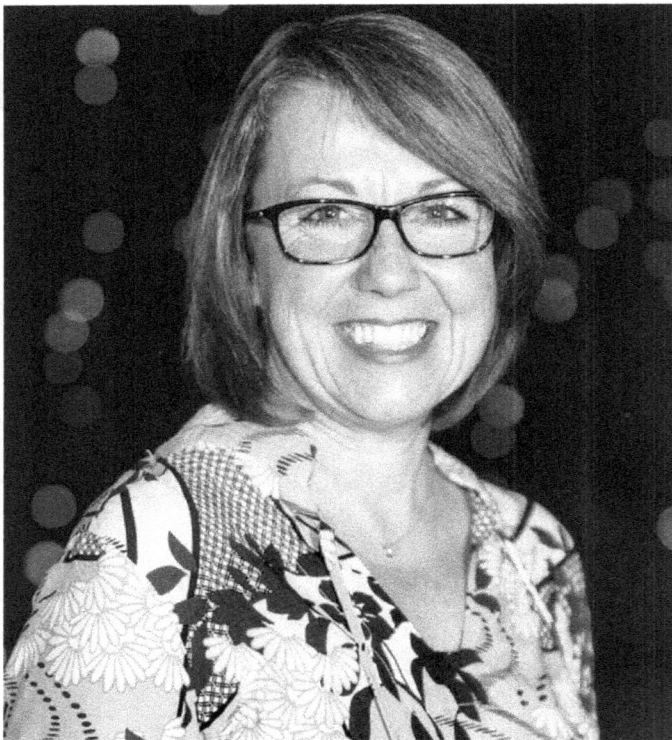

Fourteenth Story

By Jo Christmas

Many years ago, when I was working as a sister in a hospice, someone suggested to me that all illnesses were emotional or energetic in origin. I thought they were crazy.

It's funny how the things we sometimes reject without consideration come back and revisit us. Twenty-seven years on, I have adopted similar views and can see a certain kind of wisdom in our bodies and disease. Firstly though, I want to make a distinction between who we are as people and the diagnosis of breast cancer. You (or whoever has been diagnosed) are not the breast cancer. Each of us, whilst similar in many ways, are unique and so much more than just our physical bodies. We have all heard incredible stories of how a mother managed to lift a car just enough to pull her child from underneath, fuelled by the most incredible love. I can't tell you the number of patients I cared for who were told they only had weeks to live, and then surprised everyone by living long enough to attend their son or daughter's wedding several years later. Or the patient who was finally discharged from hospice care after having lived cancer-free for 5 years. I have been surprised and wrong so many times I've become really comfortable with not knowing. Actually, I've come to appreciate my uncertainty, because even when I have convinced myself I can't or won't be able to do something, the impossible still remains a possibility. If we've already decided an outcome, then we probably won't even try to create something different. I've noticed that we can be powerful influencers of our bodies and our life if we so choose but we have to be prepared to get up close and personal. We need to learn our bodies language; listen to its whisperings, which may come in the form of intuition, emotions and symptoms, before we can respond to its wisdom.

Ok, so if you acknowledge that you are more than a diagnosis and you are open to the possibility or like the idea of having some influence over how you are experiencing life, I want you to put that diagnosis to one side and start to see yourself (or the person diagnosed) separately. What makes you happy? What do you love to do and how do you love to feel? These are important questions we often avoid asking ourselves or believe that those choices are out of our control. Well, guess what? Now is the time! This is the gift hidden under the shock, disbelief, anger and fear of being diagnosed. It really is time to come back to you and place yourself in the centre stage. What is important to you? What do you need to think, feel, do in order to be present and happy right now? Stay with me, I know it sounds a bit out there, but sometimes a completely different perspective opens up opportunities and possibilities to us that we haven't been able to see before. As my mate Einstein says, you can't solve a problem from the same level of thinking that created it, which I interpret as meaning that it's difficult to be healthy when you are focusing on the sickness.

I had always thought of health as being something that you had (or not) as well, but now I think of health from an entirely different perspective. Rather than being a constant, I think of health and wellness being on a continuum, tipping in one direction or another dependant on how we are feeling about ourselves, what is happening in our lives and the subsequent choices we make. I believe that even the smallest change in behaviour has a consequence, and so influences the outcome. Based on my belief that illness and wellness are actually on a continuum and you have more influence over your health than you have previously been aware of, each choice you make has the potential to either move you in one direction or the other.

Whilst I don't like to make generalisations and am aware there are always exceptions, often the individuals that I met who had been diagnosed with breast cancer were incredibly nurturing and caring and it got me thinking, *Were they so busy nurturing others, that they forgot to care for themselves?* What if this diagnosis was a scream from their loving bodies to stop and take notice of what was happening within them and apply that love and nurturing they offered to others, to themselves? Sometimes when we constantly give of ourselves, we forget that we also need to take time to top up as well. That's the balancer. That's what keeps us well and allows us to continue giving from a full, healthy space.

What if the symptoms that make up illnesses and diseases are in fact our bodies' way of desperately trying to communicate important information to us, but because we are so busy and distracted from ourselves or just don't understand or like those initial subtle bodily messages we miss or ignore the information until it turns up the volume? The diagnosis of breast cancer cannot be ignored, and it makes us take notice. Now, I am not trying to trivialise anything or suggest any blame, I am wanting to highlight our point of power and ability to take charge and influence our lives. I can see how this may sound crazy to some of you, but I actually think we live in a crazy world; life is busier than it has ever been, we often eat food with little nutrition on the run, have a coffee to propel us forward when we need to stop, take medicine so we can go to work when we are so sick we should be resting up at home. We are so focused on what we "have" to do and where we "have" to go, we forget to be present to ourselves, missing how tired, stressed and overwhelmed we are. We often get pushed further and further down the line of priorities, attending to everyone and everything we think we "have" to do until we almost disappear. Now, does that sound like something you would do to someone you loved or cared about? I think in our busyness and beliefs about needing to do do do, we have forgotten how special life is, how special we are, how to care for ourselves and how to be and enjoy the present moment. Just take a moment to consider – is it possible that some of this might apply to you? If you're like me, you may worry that considering your needs is selfish, but it is not selfish to take care of ourselves. In doing so, people get best from us. It might actually be selfish not putting our needs first? I think the word selfish should be replaced with "self-full". When we are taking care of our needs, no one else has to worry about us and we get to share more of the fullness of who we are. Oh, and we get to model to those around that we care about that it is ok for them to love themselves and do what is right to keep themselves happy and healthy. Are you laughing? Thinking, *What is this girl on?*

Well, what I learned whilst working in a hospice is that life is precious and that we often don't get to realise just how precious it is until it is too late. We all come with an expiry date. I realised that even with a terminal diagnosis, that diagnosis can be the most incredible opportunity to stop and think about what is important to you, how you want to be and maybe consider how you can live more fully and joyfully in each moment. In fact, some people crammed more life into their last few months than most of us do in a lifetime. I don't ever remember hearing people saying that they wished they had worked harder or earned more money (even though money was sometimes a concern), but rather they wished they had spent more time playing with their kids rather than working, seen that sunrise, gone on that trip or just enjoyed themselves more. What an opportunity a diagnosis can be (if you let it) to take a stock check of where you are and become more active in creating what you want. Some people aren't lucky enough to have this opportunity.

Ok, so the good news is that you have a diagnosis that has got your attention. You get to think about what you want to create from now on, how you think about things and how you want to be amongst what is happening. There is no right or wrong way to think about or respond to a diagnosis of breast cancer. It's up to you. At the most basic level, you can still choose to focus on things that make you happy or you can focus on things that move you away from happiness. It might be hard initially if the diagnosis seems so big it is overshadowing you, but remember it is not you, it is a diagnosis of breast cancer.

You are so much more than that, so what makes that more-of-you happy? You may have to be really general and look at the little things if everything feels like $#*! by focusing on your breath, a blue sky, the sound of the birds, a smile from someone, the fact that you are alive right here in this moment. Why am I rambling on about this? Because what we focus on grows. I'm not suggesting you ignore the diagnosis or pretend it isn't happening, but I am suggesting that you don't make it bigger and more frightening than it already is.

Ok, so for those of you who like a bit of science, there is a whole heap of it to support how emotions can affect our health and how we move ourselves in the direction of wellness.

Each of us have a different experience of the world. Even if the events were the same, we think different thoughts, feel different emotions and have a different biological make up. We and our biology are affected by intangible elements like beauty and love, we experience emotions such as joy, excitement and bliss as well as anger, sadness and fear, and our thoughts can trigger certain emotions whether based on fact or not. Depending on which thought has been chosen, it can create anxiety as easily as joy. Our bodies react to these sometimes subtle and invisible thoughts, emotions and experiences in a very physical way by altering blood pressure and cortisol levels in an attempt to prepare itself to respond to what may occur. As we relax, we activate our parasympathetic nervous system which allows our blood pressure to lower and our cortisol levels to decrease, and we naturally breath more deeply as our bodies decide it is safe to take the time to digest food, sleep and repair. Conversely, when we think a thought that triggers a fear or makes us anxious, our bodies prepare for action; becoming alert, stopping any non-essential functions such as digestion or repairs, and focusing on keeping itself alert for any threats. Our bodies are amazing, so wise, so adaptable and always trying to create balance amongst the changes it encounters. I am in awe of its infinite intelligence, we just have to learn to take notice and work with our bodies wisdom, rather than against it.

Each thought, emotion, experience has an effect on our bodies physiology, so maybe it is not quite so surprising that these less tangible parts of ourselves also have an effect on our health.

I'm inviting you to consider how you might become more involved in caring and nourishing yourselves. I believe that we have far more power over reclaiming our health than we think, although if we are to reclaim in that power, I do think it requires a very different way of thinking and being. I want to redefine health as balance and that you will know whether your body and life are in balance depending on how you feel rather than an intellectual check list. I know this is a different way of viewing things, but I invite you to consider this possibility with curiosity, using your own observations, personal experience and wisdom rather than just your or someone else's intellect. I'll tell you why. Only you can know what is right for you. No one else has the constant feedback that you get from your body to tell you whether you are on track.

The truth is that we cannot always control what happens to us, but we can control our response. In order to be able to really influence our health and lives, we need to get to know ourselves well enough to successfully notice those little clues and subtle messages our body gives us before the crash happens. By becoming consciously aware of our thoughts, feelings and bodies, we get to notice when we are beginning to go off track as well as noticing when we feel happy, vibrant and well in ourselves and consciously direct ourselves towards more of what we want.

Self-care is so important. There is only one of you, and there will never be anyone quite like you again. No-one is in a better position to know what is in your best interests than you, however well-meant or well qualified. It's your job to really get to know and appreciate yourself, quirks and all. You can only do this by making time for yourself and really noticing who you are; what you are thinking, what you dream about, what your intuition is telling you, your feelings and what effects them, what you find yourself doing and which of those bits make you happy and fulfilled. Happy, bliss, peace, fun, love, joy, interest, clarity are good indicators you're on track. Sadness, anxiety, fear, confusion and feeling stuck might indicate a movement away from where you want to be.

Many people think about self-care in terms of a having a massage, a lovely bath, or treating yourself to something you've wanted, which are wonderful things to do for yourself, but I think it is much more fundamental than that. It's about being, rather than having to do anything. I think real self-care is about making time to be with yourself, listen and take notice of what comes up for you and to care more about how you FEEL rather than what others think about you. Then work out what is needed in this moment for you to feel more connected, happier and peaceful. We all deserve to feel good and be happy, but nobody else can do it for us, because no one else knows what it is that we need to fulfil us.

Our job is to stay present to ourselves and become our own BFF by noticing how we feel, trusting that internal wisdom and using it as our sat-nav to constantly realign ourselves in the direction of happiness, peace, love and support.

The truth is that none of us really know what the future holds, but by focusing on what may or may not happen then, we miss the opportunity to make the most of what is available to us right here, right now.

Whilst the many potentials of the future can be lived in your head, real life can only be truly experienced or influenced in the now. It is each moment that provides the opportunity for magic and meaning in life, so I invite you to be present and notice what is happening for you, then take that information and move closer to what you want to create for yourself. How would you 'be' if you were happy and vibrantly healthy; what would you be doing, thinking, how would you be feeling? Make that your point of focus. If you are off track from that point, change what you are doing, thinking, feeling to align with how you would be when you are happy and vibrantly healthy.

I've sort of come to appreciate those uncomfortable feelings such as anger, frustration or anxiety (even if it takes me a while to get there) because they remind me that I'd slipped off course. I had somehow lost myself in everything that was happening and needed to refocus on what I needed to nourish myself and make me happy. No wonder it felt painful. The crazy thing is that those things are always there, I just stopped paying attention to them for a while and forgot that it is my responsibility to love and care for myself and that there is nobody is better qualified to do this for me.

Jo Christmas is a Holistic Counsellor, Life, Health and wellness Coach. She has 2 beautiful children and lives in a bayside suburb north of Brisbane, Australia.

She has 18 years' experience as a nurse and specialised in the areas of Palliative Care, HIV/AIDS and Occupational Health.

Jo has an honours degree in Psychology, as well as a diploma in Clinical Nutrition and a diploma in counselling and is passionate about health and wellness.

You can reach Jo at jochristmas17@gmail.com.

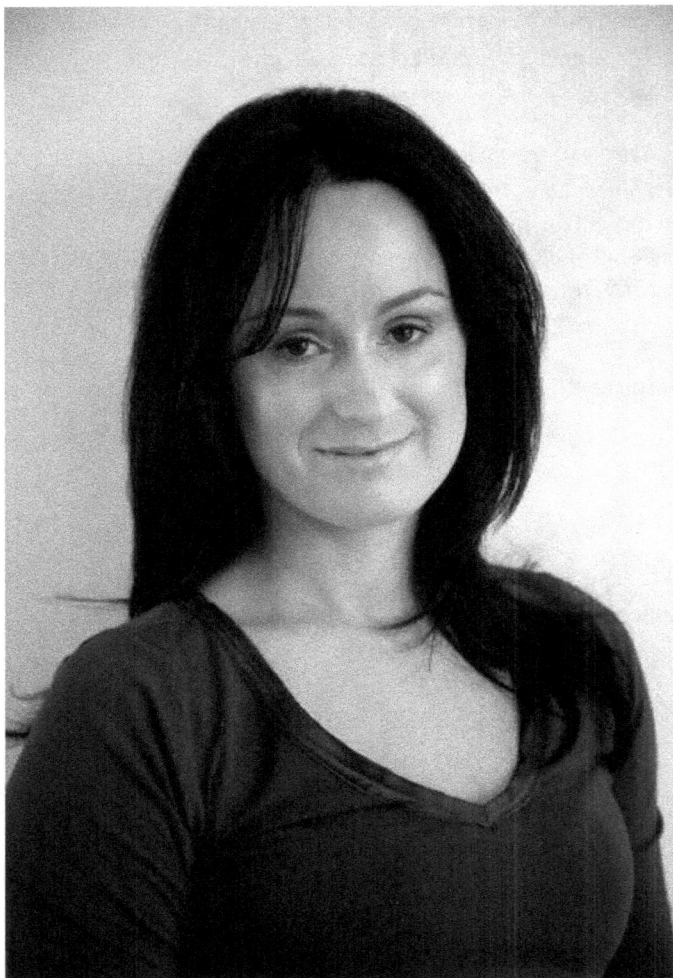

Fifteenth Story

By Haley Williams

Lots of people are time poor these days, and Sundays are precious.

I get it.

I've always loved to help. It makes me feel good. I've volunteered, run in fun-runs and favoured baby showers in support of a charity over gifts. So my latest "brunch" left me feeling a bit sad.

You see, a year ago, my mum was diagnosed with breast cancer. It was the darkest few months of my life, and it shocked me how quickly life can be turned on its head. How lonely and isolating it is to have someone you love face such a disease. If ever I was afraid, my mum was my first confidant. No longer could I confide in her about what was the greatest fear I've ever felt in my life.

What surprised me most was the hopelessness that wedged itself in my heart and wouldn't let go. Not to let me sleep, or enjoy my children, or even to eat or participate in things I used to enjoy. My life just stopped in the panic and despair that only someone who has been diagnosed with cancer or has had someone close to them go through it will understand.

Waiting on results was torture. How bad was it? How far had it spread? The terror at the thought of losing my mum or what she'd have to go through was suffocating. Luckily, the results couldn't have been better. She was stage 1 (in situ) which meant surgery, a full mastectomy with no chemotherapy, was all the treatment she would need to be in the clear. The relief of this news was sweeter than the birth of my own children!

It was during my mum's surgeries that I met the wonderful women behind the Chicks in Pink charity. They were amazing and it only heightened my enthusiasm for fundraising. I saw firsthand how important this charity is to women touched by breast cancer. There were so many services offered, and extraordinary support. It was overwhelming. Obviously, it became a charity close to my heart. I'll never forget the day mum and I ran in the Chicks in Pink fun run. We crossed the line together and I could have cried. It felt so good to have done something so positive together for a charity we'd become so reliant upon and to give back.

So, it wasn't long before the Breast Ever Brunch fundraiser caught my eye and I decided to host in honour of what my mum's been through over the past year. I'd raised money for charitable causes in the past, but they weren't personal. They hadn't touched my life directly. This was different. It was personal and it was painful. In hindsight, I realise it was too raw, too soon to be raising money for a charity that became so important to me. But I couldn't help myself. So, mum and I bought, baked and decorated like crazy and out went the invitations to our Breast Ever Brunch!

Unfortunately, it wasn't a big success. Okay, that's an understatement – it bombed! Of the 20 people we invited, only four people came to brunch. It wasn't what we were expecting, but it did turn out to be a lovely morning with delicious food (lots of!) and good friends and we did raise almost $200 for a great cause.

Our feelings were hurt because it didn't turn out the way we'd hoped – but it was the way it made my friends feel, too. So many people felt bad that they couldn't come, even though I tried to reassure them that it was fine and things pop up. It was personal to us, but it wasn't like that for everyone invited.

So, in future, I won't ever put myself in a position where other people feel pressure to be part of something – especially when it's so personal – but I'll still support this important charity, in fun runs or simply making donations when I can.

Haley Williams has a Bachelor of Communication in Journalism and over a decade of experience in the media, marketing and communications industries.

She is a widely published journalist with a particular interest in writing magazine features on parenting, health, fitness, nutrition and education.

Before becoming a freelance journalist, Haley worked as a writer for NeoLife (a worldwide nutrition company), News Limited and APN News & Media.

Haley also has extensive experience as an SEO Content Writer and Digital Marketing Strategist.

@HaleyWilliams – Twitter

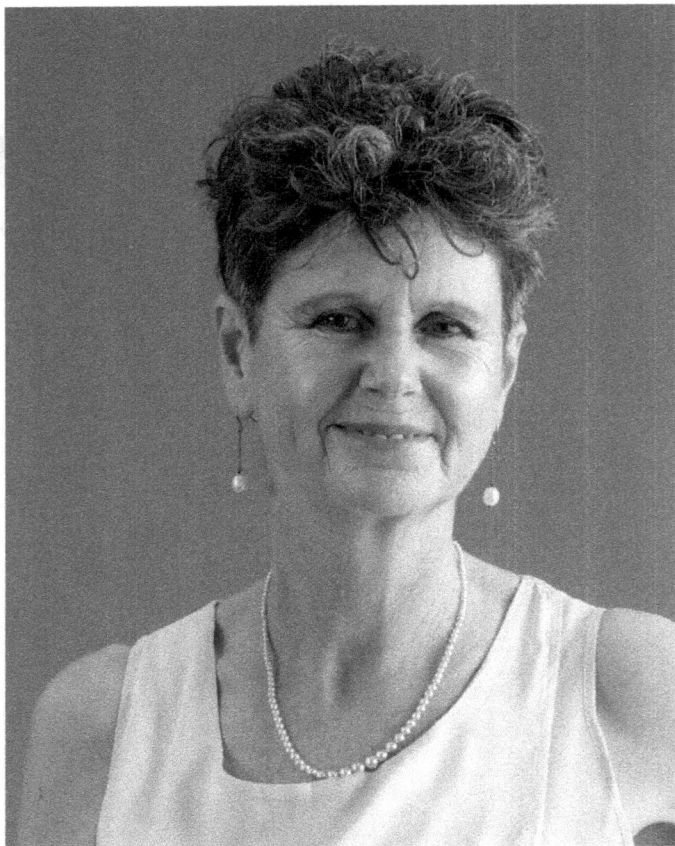

Sixteenth Story

By Julie Brand

"Cancer care today often provides state-of-the-science biomedical treatment but fails to address the psychological and social problems associated with the illness." - excerpt from *Cancer Care for the Whole Patient: Meeting Psychosocial Health Needs*

Boy, did that resonate when I read it!

This is the story of my breast cancer experience and its aftermath.

I knew nothing about breast cancer. I didn't even know there were two t's in the word mastectomy 'till I had one! Slowly though, I have had to learn all about breast cancer. I had a reconstruction that started on the same day as the mastectomy, but that reconstruction didn't end well. After seven months I asked my plastic surgeon to "just take it out, please". So, she did. Following that failure, my only option for a normal looking bust was to use an external breast prosthetic. So, I duly went where I was told to go and bought this awful thing! I thought, 'I can't possibly wear this for the rest of my life!' And I wouldn't, so I made my very own.

My partner Franco Pierucci and I decided to establish a company that remains the only one in Australia making external breast prostheses for women who have a breast as I have. It's called "Perfect Again" because even if you didn't really like your breasts, once they are gone, you realise that, actually, they really **were** perfect!

We imported a robotic machine that uses scanning technology. We are able to scan a woman's post-operative chest landscape, which of course is unique to her alone, and then scan the shape of her remaining breast. These two scans are married together in a cad cam program, which in turn drives our clever robotic carving machine to make a simple, two-part mould which we use to make that particular woman's breast form.

Simple!

After doing this for about a hundred women and learning lots of stuff, we realised that we'd have to make a range of ready-to-wear breast forms as well... and these are the game-changers!

There are 14 sizes in this range of breast forms – from a 32B to a 46EE – and they come in a right-hand and left-hand side version. Every breast form size also comes with two different inside contours, and most (like 88%) women who have bought them are entirely satisfied by them and will buy them again in another two years!

Gotta love that!

They cost $400 each, which is refunded by Medicare. Getting the Medicare rebate was surprisingly easy, as a matter of fact. I simply informed Medicare about the business we were about to commence, and now I email Medicare the invoice with our letterhead and the client's completed Medicare form, and $400 is refunded to an Australia woman every two years per breast form required.

Our breast forms are totally different form the old generation of heavy breast forms. They are lightweight and really comfortable. You can swim in them and once again (or perhaps for the very first time) wear beautiful bras! They are a drop-dead easy solution and are WAY cheaper and safer than a reconstruction! If, indeed, you eventually want to have a reconstruction, they are a great way to look normal whilst waiting for everything to settle down, both inside and outside of your head before you have that hard-core breast reconstruction.

It launched in February 2014. I wanted a better external breast prosthesis than the weighted one I had to buy back in 2002, and I thought that perhaps all the women of Australia would buy one too. It seemed like such a good idea at the time — indeed, the whole idea was brimming with potential...

How naive were we?

Establishing then running a successful business is surely the hardest thing to do in the whole wide world! If Franco and I knew then what we know now, there is NO WAY that we would have even tried it! I can only conclude that we were completely insane!

We used the wrong marketing people to the tune of many thousands of dollars, and yet I remain a TERRIBLE marketing person who will never be able to successfully market our breast forms! Half a million dollars is DEFINITELY not enough to make a successful business of breast forms in Australia!

The medical arena in which we now find ourselves is VERY conservative, and our breast forms are so revolutionary that no medicos want to touch them or us, even though 88% of our clients are entirely satisfied with our them!

Word-of-mouth really is the best recommendation – but it's SO slow! Girl friends don't get breast cancer together! We get it one by one. So, you can't even tell your best friend about this fabulous product you've just found!

And we've learned more stuff...

1.   We've learned that women put up and shup up.

They assume the "burnt chop" attitude to life. This means that they, almost without exception, at a barbecue give the best chops to their kids, then they'll give the second-best chops to their husbands, and finally, they will eat the burnt chops themselves. This simply illustrates that women put themselves and their comfort way behind everyone else's wellbeing in their family.

2.   Women who have recently had a breast cancer diagnosis are preyed upon by many self-interested parties.

There are the female sellers of weighted breast forms (who have never needed to wear one) who make pronouncements and predictions that will have major impacts on the quality and comfort of a woman's future life based purely on selling product.

3. There are some medicos who want a woman to immediately embark upon a reconstruction (at about 20k per breast), which are called "recons" in the trade. Let's hope these women are also told all the downsides of these "recons" as well!

These downsides include the "no guarantee of a good outcome", or the 20k per breast reconstruction, that it will always feel weird. Or that a reconstruction will take many long operations, and even then, you may not like the outcome. Or that the reconstructed breast will move and or change shape and size. (If you wish to embark on a reconstruction, please seek and ask other women who have done this before and be advised by their first-hand experience.)

Remember that a reconstructed breast using plastic surgery will NEVER give you back your lost breast and you can't take it out at night...

4. I would recommend that a woman at the very least, **pauses** between her breast surgery and any reconstruction she may wish to undertake.

5. Breast cancer is a very great trauma physically and mentally and often takes five long years to fully recover! Yes, I know that a sound terrifying but it's true and it happened to me!

6. But, women endure, and we overcome ... it all takes time!

We women are looked after beautifully medically during our time of breast diagnosis, surgery and the therapies that follow. But, perhaps, we could be helped more emotionally during this time, because it is one of the most difficult and traumatic times of our lives.

Women should be counselled to really look into themselves to work out the best way for them personally to recover. Take learning, for example: every single person learns quite differently. Likewise, every single person recovers quite differently. We should be guided into thinking about and deciding on which way is the best way for us to recover. Then we can confidently walk towards our recovery, which actually will make it easier and faster.

Perfect Again will proceed until Christmas 2018. Franco and I will assess everything then and decide what to do at that point. However, we can't keep pushing water uphill forever!

Julie Brand – Director of Perfect Again Breast Forms.

She established this business because she had to use one of the old-generation heavy breast forms following her own mastectomy back in 2002.

Perfect Again Breast Forms are loved by 88% of the women who wear them because they are lightweight and comfortable, and you can forget you're wearing one.

They are worn with beautiful bras, too.

Perfect Again's Breast Studio is located at Portarlington, regional Victoria, but they sell and ship our products all over Australia.

For all further information, please call Julie on (03) 5259 1919 or 0408 502 344.

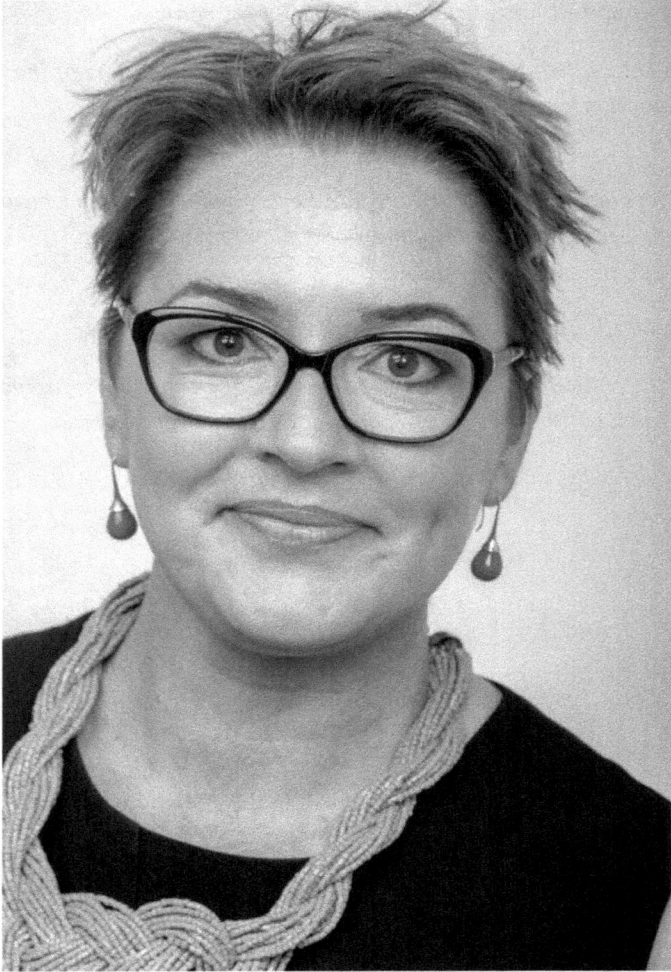

Seventeenth Story

By Kylie Warry

Facing a family legacy.

It's funny – when you are well, you don't even notice that you are well. You just take advantage of the fact that you can do whatever you decide to do in the moment. I can remember those days if I look back now.

I remember silly little things like, walking around a shopping centre all day, like finishing work and thinking, 'Let's go to the movies.' I remember not recoiling when my husband touched me.

I'm 45, and I was diagnosed with breast cancer at 41. There is a strong family history. I am one of 4 girls, and I am the youngest. My mum died after a 30+ year fight with breast cancer and my sister has had a double mastectomy – a year after mum died. I have aunts and cousins who have had and died from breast cancer. We do not have the BRCA gene but have been told we have a yet unidentified gene due to the recurrence and age of the women in my family when diagnosed.

The story I want to share is as much about my Mum as it is about me, because my early experience with breast cancer shaped the woman I became. Living with this dreadful disease looming over my head indeed shaped me more than I realised at first.

It was always my biggest fear growing up that I would lose my Mum before I was ready (when are you ever ready??). I was 31 when she did lose her battle, I still didn't feel ready.

My Mum was diagnosed with breast cancer when I was just a baby and she was breast feeding. She found the lump but it was thought to be a mastitis infection, so it was ignored for a while. Eventually she persisted, and it was found to be cancer. I had no idea; I was just a baby.

My first memory was going to doctor appointments with her, and her being really afraid. I don't think looking back that I really knew what was going on. I just knew she was scared, and I felt like I was looking after her, making sure she felt safe. A very big job for a little girl.

Mum had a mastectomy when I was a toddler. I didn't know what this meant, but I saw the prosthetic she would put in her bra. I used to play with it as a little girl; she called it her chicken fillet. I don't remember Mum getting upset with me for playing with it. I hope I didn't say or do anything that was embarrassing for her.

The first time I remember fearing my Mum may die was when I was about 7. Mum was out for the evening and was late coming home. I was still up and I remember having this feeling of dread, and not knowing why. The phone rang, and we were told Mum had been in a car accident.

My dad, sister and I jumped in the car and drove to the site of the accident. As we got there, my dad and sister made me stay in the car and left me while they went to Mum at the accident site. All I could see was crumpled cars, flashing lights, and I saw mum being put into an ambulance. I lost it, I was screaming and trying to fight my way out of the car, but I too scared to leave the vehicle.

The fear I felt then is still tangible today, such an awful memory. The accident ended up being a blessing as mum hurt her back, and when they did scans they found the cancer had metastasized to her spine. She was placed on Tamoxifen, and I am not sure of the other treatment except for radiation. She always had pain, I never understood why. Later I would understand more fully.

Life went on. I was a busy kid; I realise now that I was a chronic over achiever; I think that in my own journey to self-discovery I learned that my way of trying to fill this awful void, this fear of loss was to become the best at anything I tried. It seemed to work for a while, until it didn't...

I also realise now that I became a perfectionist, my way of trying to control things around me when everything felt out of control. Fearing that any day I could lose my Mum did that to me. It was only as an adult that I realised my daily battle with perfectionism and anxiety.

When I was 16 and beginning the HSC, Mum was told to stop the Tamoxifen as they were not sure of the long-term effects. A few months later, she found a lump in her remaining breast. She told her GP, who said to her, "Surely it couldn't be," and, "Not to worry!" Again, she had to push and fight to be heard – they found another tumour in her remaining breast. I sat through the HSC while my Mum went through her second mastectomy and more radiation. She was put back on Tamoxifen.

She was such a trooper. Yes, she was in pain, she ached all over, she really struggled with anxiety, but she didn't complain. I never heard her complain. In some ways, I wonder if I supported her enough, because she was always so "ok" that I just didn't think it was as big a deal as it really was. As it does, life went on...

When I was 23 and about to get married, Mum was diagnosed with an aortic aneurysm and needed emergency surgery. Both Mum and Dad couldn't be at my wedding as she was in the middle of the most critical surgery of her life.

I remember feeling so sad that they weren't going to be there, but Mum made me promise not to postpone the big day. We went and stayed with them a couple of weeks after the wedding and Mum was again stoic, but in so much pain.

Again, she was told by her GP to stop the Tamoxifen, it had been 5+ years, so she did. One of my sisters who was a nurse was concerned as she felt she noticed a pattern – each time the Tamoxifen was stopped, the cancer seemed to resurface.

Within a few months Mum, was actually speaking of her hip pain, which was unusual. She went to the GP and for months asked for help with the pain. She eventually was sent to a specialist, where she said that she feels like her hip is broken. The cocky young registrar said, "You'd know it if you were walking on a broken hip."

But he didn't know my Mum... they x-rayed, and her hip was broken and riddled with cancer. Mum then needed a hip replacement.

She got through that as she always did, and by now was looking like a poor little rag doll that had been cut open and sewed back together so many times. She'd been given some reconstructive surgery for her breast but it was an awful job, poor love.

By 29, Mum found the cancer was spreading, and nothing they did could stop it. Each time she had radiation she was in so much pain; she would describe this never-ending burning. The cancer was in her liver and also in her brain.

During all of this, my Dad had become her carer – not a role he expected, but one he rose to. Mum was not an easy patient; she did not want to be a burden. My Dad had always been as fit as a bull, but like many of his generation had developed type 2 diabetes in his late 50's. In 2000, my Dad was told by his GP he needed to start walking regularly to fend off any side effects of the diabetes.

My Dad is very much like me, very black and white. He started walking every day but developed this awful pain in his hip. He saw physio's, had massages, saw specialists, and no one could work out what was going on.

In December 2000, I was pregnant with my first child, and found out that Dad also had cancer. They discovered he had such a hole in his hipbone that they could not believe he was still walking. On further investigation, the cancer was everywhere and we lost Dad within 10 weeks.

Mum battled on for another 15 months before she finally let go. You know, she was so cranky that Dad beat her to the finish line, she never got over the fact that he died before she did.

While my parents were "dying", our family rallied together and cared for both Mum and Dad at home. They both did not want to die in a hospice somewhere alone, so they died with dignity surrounded by love in their own home.

In the midst of all of this my marriage imploded. It wasn't a quick thing – I realised within the first few years of marriage that my husband had a drinking problem. He would not admit it, and it seemed the more successful we became, either in our careers, personally or financially, the more he began to unwind.

I left my marriage after Dad had passed away and while Mum was at her most unwell. I had my son who was about 18 months old, and we became such a team, spending most weekends in the Hunter Valley caring for my Mum to give my sister a break. By this time, Mum was living with my sister as she needed 24-hour support.

We did this for a year before Mum lost her fight. Within the next 12 months, my sister who had been caring for her was also diagnosed with breast cancer. She was so thankful that Mum was not alive to know as she would have blamed herself, even though, "how can we?"

I divorced in 2003, just after losing Mum. A year later I met a wonderful man, and we married in 2006. We had a blended family together her with his 2 gorgeous kids and me with my son. Life was great, full on; I was in my own business by then, and still the silent perfectionistic overachiever.

Looking back, I don't think I ever allowed myself to stop and even just feel what had happened to me. My response is when things get tough, I work harder, and little did I know, all of this would catch up with me.

I remember for at least 12 – 18 months before I was diagnosed I had felt tired, run down, and everything ached. However, I put it down to me being soft, and I just needed to "suck it up, princess". If I didn't do it, who would?

Yet, this fight got harder and harder, and pushing through was no longer an option. So, I went to see my GP. I was tired (exhausted, if I'm honest), a little over weight, (about 8 kg), unhappy with myself and I felt like I was ready to snap.

I asked for a thyroid test (in my research, I felt I had every symptom of hypothyroid). My GP refused to test me and said she would look at my iron… real helpful. I left feeling like such a whiner and thankfully I called a girlfriend. She said, "That isn't good enough your GP should listen, why don't you try this GP I've heard she is brilliant."

I made an appointment, she heard my history and was extremely thorough. I felt heard. We did a routine mammogram and ultrasound, as well as every other test known to man, including my thyroid.

At the mammogram, I felt like it was a waste of time, this was not going to be my story. I didn't even think about the possibility, but as they kept going over this one area, man it hurt! I felt like my nipple was being squeezed through a mincer.

Then the ultrasound, he was such a lovely guy, we chatted about life, love and the universe until, again, he stopped at a certain area. He stopped chatting, and I grew suspicious. I asked, "Hey, is everything ok?" He said, "I think you've booked yourself in for a biopsy, love." My head started racing. Surely not,

not me,

not now...

I can't have cancer...

That was 4 years ago. I am better. I have had a double mastectomy, chemotherapy and hormone therapy. I live daily with chronic fatigue (some call it post-chemo fatigue). The chemo has wreaked havoc on my immune system with me dealing with uncontrolled Hashimoto's Thyroiditis (yes, I did have a thyroid issue, too), and it looks like I am developing more autoimmune conditions.

I am coming to terms with the battle my body and I went through (and are still going through). I am no longer the same woman I was pre-cancer. It changes you, for the better and for the worse. I am working on accepting my new body and how it feels. I am shifting from the idea that my body is broken, to a more loving thought: "My body is a warrior that has been to hell and back; it's battle worn, has scars, but has a wisdom and a strength beyond words."

This journey is hard, gut wrenching and life changing. I encourage you though, look for the gifts. Look for the learning and the messages for you. For me, it was to appreciate myself. To stop "doing" for everyone else and to "just be" for me. I was last on my list for such a long time, and now I am working on being much higher up, if not first (that's a hard one for any woman or mum).

I am learning to deal with perfectionism and choose progress over perfection. A wonderful change... I am also learning to deal with the anxiety that was carved out in my childhood and stayed as an unhelpful overprotective friend.

Cancer taught me to look after me. To stop trying to be everything for everyone else. To stop expecting perfection from myself as this is never going to happen, I am already enough just as I am. The beautiful thing is, so are you...

People can chat to Kylie via her blog
http://baldbarrenandboobless.com or email kylie@kyliewarry.com.

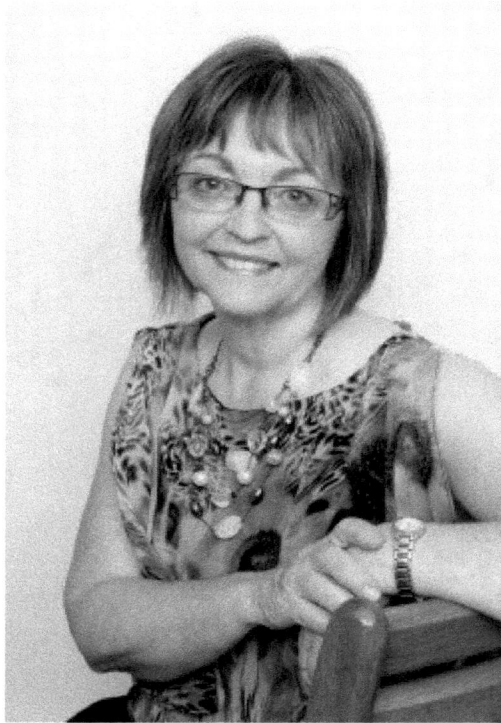

Eighteenth Story

By Marney Perna

Breast Cancer planted a seed!

In my early teens, from around 10 years of age, our family faced many years of financial hardship, disarray and health calamities. During a family visit to my uncle's farm, dad had a farming accident. He was pitching in to help out, and his right hand became lodged in an onion grader. Thanks to the very quick work on my cousin's part in stopping the tractor immediately, it wasn't more severe than it was. However, his hand was stuck in the machine and my uncle didn't have the knowledge to get it out. My dad had to instruct my uncle on how to dismantle the machine. The ambulance took forever to arrive, and little did we children know it or understand it, but our lives had changed for ever.

Dad was a fitter and turner and worked with his hands. He had just started a new job, so suddenly there was no income, no insurance, no sick leave, and our home was a rented housing commission house. Fifty plus years ago, there was no such thing as real charity or government assistance. Because dad was helping my uncle, he didn't qualify for workers compensation, even if my uncle had it at the time, which he didn't! They were also not able to help mum and Dad in any way, so we had to get out of the mess ourselves.

Here we were, a family with four children under 11, in a rented house, no income and no family support. When mum approached the government for some assistance, they tried to take the two younger children into care! Mum chased them out of the house with a broom! Some things remain in your memory as clear as day!

So, mum got a job doing night fill, and one night a large tin of Pal dog food dropped on her chest, causing severe pain and bruising. The next day, she went to see the doctor. After a comprehensive check, mum was told she had suspected breast cancer and to prepare for the possibly of not living for many months longer! With no one to turn to, family too busy in their own lives, husband still in hospital facing numerous operations and rehabilitation.

Total shock, so mum set about ensuring that we could become resilient children and could cope on our own... she showed us how to cook a three-course meal comprising of tinned soup, basic meat and vegies and a pudding with tinned fruit, self-saucing pudding, etc. We learned to help out in the house and to share the jobs around. At the time, we were renting a three-bedroom housing commission home at Redbank, on the outer skirts of Brisbane. There was not a lot of assistance in those days, and mum and dad fought hard to keep the family together. Dad sold our car, and a trailer that he had been building. We were all too young to fully realise what was going on, although we did know the stress the family unit was under.

Mum went into the operation and was told afterwards that her breasts were filled with lots of little fatty tissue lumps and cysts and that she would have to be very careful of from then on. Although she was pleased to find out that it wasn't cancer, it had caused considerable trauma in our family unit. Mum had horrible scarring from the operation and always carried the "emotional trauma scar" of that episode in her life. Now, as an adult, I still find it very hard to comprehend and understand the enormity and isolation mum and dad must have found themselves in. Their resilience and tenacity was remarkable.

So, the C seed was planted.

Many years later, mum's eldest sister, Aileen, was diagnosed with a severe and aggressive form of breast cancer. Auntie Aileen was a nun and a very private and gentle woman. Her cancer was a fast, aggressive, nasty form of cancer. It was very difficult for her emotionally and she found the physical side of it very confronting as well. She was used to privacy, and those who have travelled the cancer journey know there is no privacy or delicacy involved. Mum, myself and my baby daughter became her support buddies. We travelled together to surgeries, doctor visits and copious chemo trips. We supported her practically and mentally, although her pure faith and conviction of a God's Plan gave her hope and serenity. There was still the shock of diagnosis, the utter disbelief that it was happening and, for the two sisters, the worry of leaving each other.

For my mum, it also bought back many feelings of another time and place that was starting to pile up and gnaw at her confidence.

Auntie Ail also lost her hair fairly quickly. She often commented that being a nun had her well trained for having no hair as in the early days of being in a religious order they had to shave their head to be able to wear a veil. However, she mentioned that this was different, and her head got very sore and painful. So, we found a pattern and made copious soft material caps. We made them to match her outfits, so that she felt very trendy and uplifted. She would also share them with others who didn't have anyone to make them. During those years of caring for my aunt I saw firsthand the resilience and day to day fortitude that cancer patients needed to be able to cope. The enormous emotional trauma a diagnosis and subsequent treatment took on the health and wellbeing of them. It affected and permeated into family, friends and communities. The stories we listened to from others on their own journey, whilst sitting through long days of chemo sessions, the amazing care and concern given by the nursing staff and the ups and downs of life were indeed both heart breaking and heartening at the same time. I also noticed that many women had no support, from family or communities, and I often wondered how they coped.

My aunt passed from breast cancer and it left a big hole in our family. It was in those following days that I realised that although the person had passed, the remaining family members were still strangely caught up in the threads left behind by the fight and emotional connections that are a big part of cancer. I also came to understand the fortitude and resilience shown by those travelling their own cancer journey. It is a very personal journey and not always able to be shared or carried by others. Such is the nature of cancer.

The C seed had sprouted and grown!

Several years passed and I met and knew many women of all ages diagnosed with breast cancer or the threat of breast cancer. I became a regular visitor to the Wesley Breast Clinic both in support of others or as a recipient of preventative mammograms and clinic visits. When one has had a close family member experience breast cancer it adds to the possibility of being diagnosed personally. One of my friends had a predisposition to develop cysts and had to be closely monitored. She also was unable to drive for her check-ups, so a group of her close friends including myself used to make a group booking for our regular check-ups. Afterwards we would go to a lovely café and all breathe a sigh of relief that we were asked to come back next year… until, that was, one of our group got the shocking diagnosis of "we have found a lump!"

The Wesley Breast Clinic is a place of raw and high emotions, anxiety, relief and trauma. It is generally filled with women of all ages, sizes, races and religions attempting to stay calm and positive whilst being wrapped in a gown that didn't always fit comfortably. Knowing that the mammogram would be uncomfortable and awkward, but always hoping against hope that you got to get the right coloured slip to then be able to get dressed and go home. However, many times you had to have a further mammogram or ultrasound as they eliminated a possible challenge, then you might also have to see the resident doctor. On those occasions your heart sank, and if it was a friend you often felt a bit of selfish guilty relief that it was not you getting the same further checks. The fact that all these services could be offered whilst attending that appointment did however make it easier, especially if you had travelled some distance to have the check-up. The staff and care workers were lovely and always mindful of the emotions and situations of the women there. They made a scary place less scary.

Our group of four suddenly became a group of three as one of the friends went from "see you in a year" to her own ongoing cancer journey. She always said how lucky and fortunate she was to have found it as a small seed and not an advanced tumour. She has now passed her 10-year mark cancer free. A year on, another of our group was also diagnosed with a possible cancer diagnosis, and she also had to have further ongoing treatment and sessions. Suddenly, there were two! You can imagine how extremely nervous and anxious we both were at our next annual check-up! The sigh of relief and exultation was amazing when we both got to go home.

The C seed was flowering!

I am a natural therapist and have seen many clients who have experienced their own cancer journey, some with breast cancer and some with cancer in other parts of their body. They come to see me for support for the stress and emotional trauma a diagnosis gives, and they are also looking for hope of the future. The shock of a cancer diagnosis for either the person or their family can rock people to the very core of their inner harmony; the stress and continual effects of the stress of treatment can overload the immune system and put even more strain on the adrenal systems. It can leave them vulnerable to further complications and ill health. Sometimes, it makes them feel totally disconnected from themselves and unable to foresee or have hope for a better future.

It is important to support someone with words of encouragement and empowerment. Nearly everyone knows someone or knows of someone who had fought with the big C. The journey, the end result or even the treatment is not the same for everyone, however I have noticed that most people love to share the story of the worst-case scenarios, and when initially coming to terms with a diagnosis you do not wish to hear all the sad tales.

One of processes I use in my clinic is language intention. That is to use language that is of a higher vibration and energy, a word that uplifts or doesn't add to the shock that is already being experienced. I help people to stop giving themselves further aftershocks each time they are asked how they are or what is wrong with them! I get them to rename the condition and call it "recnac" or give it a nickname. Recnac is cancer spelt backwards, and when someone asks you what is wrong they generally do not recognise the name, so are less inclined to tell you all about everyone else's journey. It stops you having to constantly explain and acknowledge what's happening; it gives you pause from aftershocks and a moment's peace to regroup. Several of my clients also give their breasts a name, and I know one lady who threw a breast removal party. She used humour and laughter to help lighten her load. Again, it is very personal and private and up to the individual to know how to cope best for themselves. My aunt used prayer and meditation to help herself find some inner peace.

The use of quality essential oils to help alleviate pain or nausea is another option. Smell is one of our body's highest and most unique senses. Our olfactory sense is a highly tuned part of our emotional (limbic) region of our brain and can be useful to provide positive anchors from shock. One of my clients personally found the topical application of Frankincense essential oil helped to alleviate some of her physical pain, and the smell from diffusing it also assisted her to feel calmer. Each person will have their own particular scent that they like above others. Use them in nurturing baths or in diffusers or even on a hankie so that you can easily reach it when required. Play around with an assortment and verity of scents, until you connect emotionally with one.

"Hope" is yet another thing to implant and envision. Give yourself permission to look for hope and a better future. It is not saying to discount reality, it is saying to look for the possibility of a solution to your challenge. When hope is taken away, one can feel annihilated and withdrawn. Look for positives in life and use uplifting memories to assist you to feel more able to cope. Some find keeping a gratitude journal helps them to be mindful and more focused on everyday feel good moments.

Live for today, plan for tomorrow, and hope for the future.

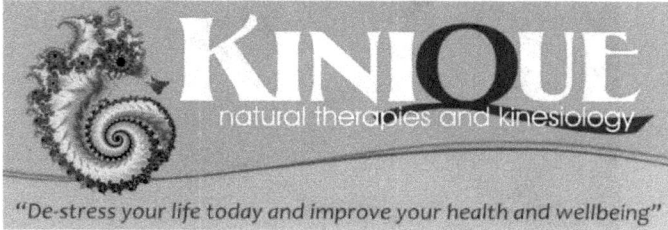

"De-stress your life today and improve your health and wellbeing"

Marney Perna
Author, Women's Health Educator and Natural Therapist
www.kinique.com

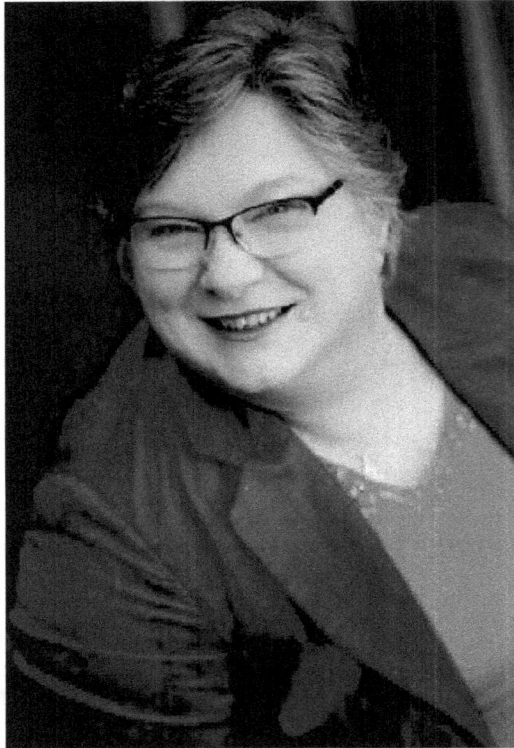

Nineteenth Story

By Janice Muir

Early in life my mother had lost her mum to breast cancer. I would have been around 4 years of age. All I can recall is that my mum was crying a lot and was in the hospital. At that point I didn't know why, but several days later I was to learn a new sister was in my life.

In my later years and with more clarity, I learned of the impact of breast cancer and some of the effects it had had on my grandmother. I recall my mother telling me when I was 12-13 years old that breast cancer was in our family and that it would skip her and one of the three of us (her daughters) would possibly be a candidate for it. I was alone with my mum when we had this conversation.

The mind is a very strong tool, it has a greater ability to conceive than we can control through our feelings and thoughts.

Life moved on. The thought was never raised again, or so I thought. In 2002, after approximately 6 years of struggle, I lost my partner to Alzheimer's dementia. I suffered a lot of stress and my eating was not balanced. Possibly one of my biggest mistakes was eating a diet of highly acidic foods prior to being diagnosed.

My daughter and I struggled. I was building a house at the time. The emotions became too much to bear, and at a point I broke down.

This story reflects my perspective and what my journey was and continues to be 10 years on. The medics predicted that I would be back in the medical system within the designated remission period of 5 years, but I defied the odds. I've lived a fairly simple life since losing my partner to Alzheimer's dementia. I sold my home and moved to Brisbane together with my daughter.

It was October 2005, when I recalled experiencing several days of bleeding between my periods. At first, I thought it was something else, but a visit to the doctor revealed symptoms of pre-cervical cancer and something needed to be done fast. I had a small operation and lost a large percentage of my cervix. The doctor recommended I take a PAP smear test annually. The news of my condition gave me a huge wake up on many levels.

I had moved houses in Jan-Feb 2006, and during this move I witnessed something very strange occur from the top of my right shoulder down to my breast. Sharp pains, a feeling of discomfort around the nipple and a piercing sensation. It was a while before I went to the doctor as the pain subsided quickly. Suddenly, in a routine personal breast assessment in the shower, I noticed something different about my breast. It was now March and I was discussing the issue seriously with my doctor. I could feel a lump in my breast. I didn't even consider that breast cancer was on the cards. It took 6 weeks to get into the medical system for my first appointment. Within days of getting into the system I had several appointments, a mammogram, a biopsy, an ultrasound and blood tests. My ultrasound result was positive, as well as my mammogram and blood test. The deciding factor was the biopsy for benign or malignant. I was a little naïve to want to accept the outcome of the X-ray or the biopsy.

I was uneasy when the radiologist on the day assured me that "This is a good hospital to be associated with, they take good care of you here." It still did not dawn on me that something was wrong. I was invincible.

The biopsy had been very painful and left me with a huge bruise. After sitting for 4-5 hours waiting for the results, the specialist stood at the door of his office to welcome me back inside where, with eyes looking into mine, he says, "There is no easy way to say this." His surgery nurse was at his side, while I was sitting alone with no one to comfort me. He proceeded to declare that the tests led to one conclusion – that I had breast cancer. By now, thoughts were running through my head... did I hear him right? How could I have this? Who was going to look after me if I was ill? I had been there for my partner, now who was going to be there for me? My only daughter was in Darwin, and my sister had her family to manage and she didn't have time to add me to her busy schedule.

A flood of emotions hit me. When it dawned on me that I was to going to need an operation I kept asking, "What operation? When? How?" I was losing it.

My daughter had lost her dad only 4 years earlier, now her mum was down with an illness that could potentially take her life.

The X-ray in front of me told me it was my name and my breast they had pictured and it had 3 lumps in it. I was given a huge number of pamphlets and after composing myself I realised I needed to drive home. I felt numb and motionless on so many levels, but I had to walk to the car to drive.

The specialist and nurse introduced me to a lovely lady called Meryl who became my support for what seemed like a huge part of the day. She was a survivor of breast cancer and it was good to have a chat with her as she was familiar with my predicament. I sat in the hospital chapel and proceeded to ring my daughter to inform her of my news. I broke down in tears as I told her. Little did I know at the time, Meryl was a volunteer at the hospital. She comforted me as we walked to the front door of the hospital. After I had consoled myself and gained some strength, I realised I would make it through. I drove home slowly, sobbing.

My biggest fear was for my daughter; how could she cope with losing both parents?

What would I do financially? I only had a temporary contract job, what would occur if I lost my job? The doctor was very compassionate and shared as much as he could on the day. Basically, I had a few days to make a decision on the date of my operation, either straight away or in three weeks' time due to public holidays.

Making a decision to operate was not easy. I had to choose between a lumpectomy or a mastectomy. I spent hours thinking about how to come to terms with this outcome. I spoke to previous breast cancer patients and did some research.

It took three weeks of spiralling up and down to reach a decision. When I was in a downward spiral, a dear close friend took my hand and asked me to "look inside the square". As I looked down at the imaginary square he pushed me backwards. I was ready to hit him, saying, "What did you do that for?" As I regained my composure he said to me, "Now take a look inside the square. You were giving up and got caught in the vortex into the hole." I was not sure; I knew I was struggling, I just did not know exactly what or where I could climb out. This proved to be a life-saver for me.

What happened for me in the next 24 hours was huge – I was able to draw out my operation to scale. My deceased partner had been a turner and fitter, and so he drew everything to scale before making it; I am a dress maker as well, and I knew how to measure and draw to scale also. This was the turning point for my decision to be made. I identified the best solution for my outcome. The next day I was due to see the doctor, and I took this paper with me to show the doctor my decision. He was amazed at the intricacy of work I had done and indicated it would be a pleasure to operate on me as he knew I was comfortable with my decision. The operation was booked for 8th of May 2006.

My journey of chemo was long and arduous. I had 8 visits every 3 weeks and 2 forms of chemo. The first knocked me out for several days and really left me flat, without the ability to do much. 4 sessions of red chemo for 3 months. The second lot of white chemo had me in a lot more discomfort – just irritation from the of loss of feeling in my feet from the last 3 months. My feet have never been the same again, especially under the toe pads. Losing the feeling in my feet during the second round of chemo had me isolated a lot more as I could not go out or drive until the last few days of the 3rd week.

My oncologist was not comfortable with my approach of taking additional vitamins during chemo, so it led me down a path of going against what the chemo specialists advised. They indicated that I would be wasting my time by taking supplements once the chemo started. This news really rocked me. My nutritionist was only too happy to research all the relevant information I had received from the hospital on my treatment and the types of chemo. We used supplements to help me cope through the whole journey.

In addition to the chemo on the 3rd week, I would visit my nutritionist who really understood food and vitamins, and he would share a way to keep the body functioning while I was on this journey. I had my blood analysed every 3 weeks with a haematologist/naturopath (the week before the next intake of chemo) and I took extra supplements and minerals.

Coming to terms with the emotions and pain I felt during the whole journey, and endeavouring to understand what was happening from this experience – the rollercoaster of tears, the new look I sported when losing my hair and what I had to do to overcome this – really had an impact on my demeanour.

I listened to positive affirmations and CDs that inspired me to keep my mind alert and focused. Every chemo session was up to 6 hours long, and I played some music that was uplifting, and also listened to motivational speakers and read personal development books for inspiration.

I played a lot of meditations and I really practiced being true to myself. I started to write a journal on several topics to keep my hand and brain in tune.

I knew some products that were designed for radiation patients and I used them daily, contrary to the medical doctor's instructions. I had faith to work it out myself and I gained the best result – I had no scar or discolouration from my radiation treatment which lasted 49 days.

I stayed with a very strong focus to succeed and come out of this a happy person. I met some lovely people along the way and they helped me stay focused after I completed treatment and was on the road to recovery. I bought a second-hand sports car, an MX5. My whole outcome changed and my focus on life became one of "go for it and live the life you can have". I followed my passion of writing and have since published a book and have others on the way. I forgave a lot of pain in my life and decided to be strong and focused in life.

My one piece of information that would benefit others on the journey... is the need to be resilient. Trust your instincts over and above the word of the doctor or the medical fraternity. Don't take everything as the truth.

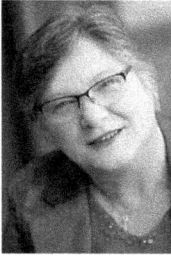

Kind regards,

Jan Muir

I Believe I Achieve

PH: 0401 009 778
EMAIL: janmuir8@bigpond.com.au
WEB: www.janmuir.com.au

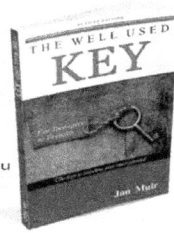

You can reach Janice Muir at her website:

www.janmuir.com.au

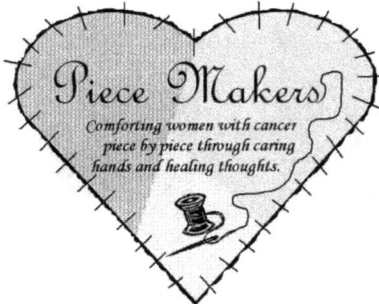

PieceMakers

You cannot help but be amazed at the generosity, both financially and of spirit, of the Caboolture and Bribie Island communities.

PieceMakers was the brain child of a Bribie resident, Laurie Griffiths, who sought to utilise her sewing talents for the good of others.

The original coordinators – Laurie, Kerry Van Schyndel and Linda Upton – met with Kim Walters Choices Program who assisted with the design and distribution of drain bags and comfort cushions which are donated to patients (in both the private and public hospitals) who have undergone surgery for breast cancer.

The benefit of these donations is twofold. Money saved by hospitals by not having to purchase these essential items, allows funds to be spent on further facilities for patients (mentoring, physiotherapy etc).

Monthly sewing meetings were originally held at Kerry's home, but eventually moved to St. Columban's College where Linda had already started a subsidiary group called StC PieceMakers, in which students of the College meet weekly after school as a co-curricular activity. Narelle Gilbert now coordinates StC PieceMakers.

Over the past 12 years, PieceMakers have donated thousands of items for distribution to patients. These are now distributed via the Wesley and St Andrew's hospitals.

Our group relies on the generous donations of materials, cottons and soft filling. If you are able to donate any of the following items, please deliver to St Columban's College for attention of PieceMakers:

- Unused cotton or cotton-blend material (not stretch) minimum 1/4m

- Cotton thread (for sewing machines or overlockers)

- Soft filling for cushions

Volunteers are always welcome.

For more information, please email piecemakersaus@outlook.com

Coordinators:
Linda Upton   0413 349 112
Narelle Gilbert 0409 057 381